Everyday Psychiatry

John Ashton
MB, BS, M.SC (SOC. MED) MRC.PSYCH, MFCM

Senior Lecturer in the Department of Community
Health at the London School of Hygiene and
Tropical Medicine.
Formerly Senior Registrar in Community Medicine,
Hampshire Area Health Authority, and Lecturer in
Community Medicine, University of Southampton

T0297246

1980
UPDATE BOOKS
LONDON/DORDRECHT/BOSTON

Available in the United Kingdom and Eire from
Update Books Ltd,
33/34 Alfred Place, London, WC1E 7DP, England

Available in the USA and Canada from
Kluwer Boston Inc.,
Lincoln Building, 160 Old Derby Street, Hingham, Mass. 02043, USA

Available in the rest of the world from
Kluwer Academic Publishers Group Distribution Centre,
PO Box 322, 3300 AH Dordrecht, The Netherlands

First published 1980
© **Update Books Ltd 1980**

British Library Cataloguing in Publication Data

Ashton, John
  Everyday psychiatry.
  1. Psychiatry
  I. Title
  616.8'9   RC454
  ISBN 0-906141-12-5

Library of Congress
Catalog Card No.: 79-67495

  Ashton, J.
    Everyday psychiatry.
  Englewood, NJ. : Update
  132 p.
  8001   790914

ISBN 0 906141 12 5

Text set in 11/12 pt Photon Times, printed and bound
in Great Britain at The Pitman Press, Bath

To my mother and in memory of my father

Contents

Preface

The idea for *Everyday Psychiatry* originated some years ago when I was working in hospital psychiatry. I had come to feel uneasy about the emphasis on traditional psychiatric teaching and practice; psychiatry somehow seemed to function in a vacuum removed from the social reality of many of the patients.

It seemed particular odd to me that psychiatrists in training were not required to spend some time in general practice so that they could obtain an understanding of the spectrum of psychiatric morbidity *and normality*. I felt that the lack of this understanding rendered a large part of psychiatric teaching irrelevant to students who were going to practise medicine in the community. In short, I felt that psychiatry was not really satisfying the needs of undergraduates and general practitioners.

A period spent in general practice and teaching undergraduates about psychiatry in general practice and the community reinforced these ideas and prompted me to start writing a series of articles, which were published in *Update*. The response to these articles was very encouraging and they have been used as a basis for *Everyday Psychiatry*.

The approach taken in this book is by nature selective and personal. The intention is to show that there is an abundance of fascinating clinical data available from psychiatry which is of immediate relevance in general practice, and that psychiatry can be a most enjoyable part of medicine.

John Ashton
Southampton, 1979

Foreword

One of the major problems of teaching or learning psychiatry is that in most medical curricula it is treated as just another subject for which time must be found in an increasingly congested programme. Its inclusion later rather than earlier in the conventional clinical course has implications for its ranking in comparison to the organ- or system-based clinical disciplines and produces a pattern of learning in which psychological insights or skills appear to be optional extras in the armamentarium of the developing clinician. The culture of hospital can also create an atmosphere in which psychiatric illness is seen either as rare, usually severe and only to be managed by referral to a psychiatrist, or simply a manifestation of personal inadequacy in patients whose problems fail to respond to conventional medical management.

Hopefully this caricature and stereotype is dated, if not already out-of-date. Students who have spent any time in general practice, as an increasing proportion do, are immediately made aware of the true prevalence of emotional and psychiatric disorder in the community and appreciate the importance of behavioural factors in the diagnosis and management of the patient in his natural environment. Students, however, may still be confused by the apparent discrepancy between experience in general practice where a large number of patients are managed by simple supportive measures or pharmacology and the apparently more complicated problems of the disturbed and often distressingly disturbed patients of psychiatric clinic or hospital. Unless psychiatric teaching has been carefully planned and integrated, the student may find it difficult to achieve a sense of perspective or to begin to appreciate and develop his own potential in the diagnosis and management of psychological disorders. This book should provide considerable help.

From a background of psychiatry, epidemiology and primary care, John Ashton has produced a book which convincingly demonstrates the contribution psychiatry can make to the understanding and management of a wide range of problems, from anxiety and depression to many which are not conventionally regarded as psychiatric in nature. Following the introductory chapter, in which he discusses the concepts of psychiatric disorder and the relationship between doctor and patient, Ashton considers individual syndromes in an epidemiological, aetiological and therapeutic framework and then explores the emotional and behavioural problems of each age of man. The problem based sections on childhood and adolescence, sexuality, drug abuse and the psychiatry of old age will be of particular value to the general practice reader. The author has achieved an effective review of the field of psychological medicine and its contribution to contemporary thought. He has successfully avoided excessive detail, but has compensated by suggesting additional reading for each chapter. In remarkably few pages he has expressed his own philosophy and demonstrated a balanced integrated approach to a wide range of problems in patient care. I hope the reader will derive as much enjoyment and benefit as I have.

Professor J. H. Walker
Department of Family and
Community Medicine
Newcastle-upon-Tyne

Acknowledgement

In writing this book, I owe a debt to my teachers and colleagues in Newcastle-upon-Tyne and Southampton and to the students who have been my guinea pigs. Any errors of commission or omission are, however, mine.

I wish to acknowledge my debt to Pam, Keir, Matthew and Nicholas who tolerated my evening absences while I was working on this book, and to Ann Harrison who typed the manuscript with such dedication.

1. Concepts of Psychiatric Disorder

In recent years a great deal of criticism has been levelled at the use of the 'medical model' in psychiatry. This has generally been by those who would like to replace it with a sociological or socioeconomic model. It is likely that any such unidimensional model would suffer from similar shortcomings to that which it replaced, and that it is only by being able to tolerate the uncertainty and ambiguity of using several models and perspectives simultaneously that we are best able to render our patients appropriate service.

In the day-to-day practice of medicine in the community, the limitations of diagnostic classifications of mental illness based on hospital populations are only too apparent. The International Classification of Disease (ICD) classification for psychiatric disorders, in its attempt to define categories which are mutually exclusive and jointly exhaustive, has resulted in a confusion between descriptive and aetiological diagnoses. It also exerts a pressure to define patients in terms of whether or not they have a condition, rather than the degree to which they have it and what relationship this bears to their previous personality and present life circumstances.

In addition to these problems, psychiatric disorders have the most severe limitation of all; they cannot be seen under a microscope, measured on an ECG or detected by the wizards in biochemistry. Much of their assessment therefore depends on the observation skills of the doctor and the ability of the patient to communicate his feelings and thoughts. The differing value systems that both doctor and patient bring to the consultation must also be considered. Again, the medical model, with its mechanistic approach to dysfunction, tends to compartmentalize and deduce, when what is so often needed is synthesis.

Similarly, the relationship between physical and emotional disorders is one of the most common difficulties in the general practice setting. Adequate assessment of physical illness always requires an understanding of what the illness means to the patient and how he feels about it. To arrive at a working model, it is necessary to look at both the doctor and the patient and then to see how they affect each other in the consultation and subsequent outcome.

The Doctor

Despite considerable changes in university admission policy, the intake of students into medical school remains one with a very narrow, middle-class base, especially people from a professional background. This, together with the lengthy and intensive training, results in the production of professional people who share a value system which differs widely from that of many of their patients. While not suggesting that doctors are standard products of a production line, it seems reasonable to take into account to what extent the background and professional training influence the way in which doctors approach their patients. In particular, the concept of the doctor 'role' is one which has some use in identifying expectations and sources of misunderstanding. This role includes the idea that doctors have internalized the behaviour and expectations of their teachers in training and that there are certain ideas about the way in which doctors should behave towards their patients and vice versa. This role also carries with it preconceptions of the nature of illness and of what people should and should not be able to cope with. It also has a tendency to carry with it a view of the consultation which, in Berne's (1964) terms, is a parent–child one. Within such a relationship, the child brings the illness to the expert (parent) who tells him what to do ('take these tablets', 'stop smoking', etc.) and the patient is supposed to do as he is told. Both parties expect the patient to get better and he usually does. If he does not, he may become labelled as a difficult patient (child) and the doctor as a poor doctor (parent). This is especially likely to happen with psychiatric problems.

Increasingly, since the war, attempts have been made in medical schools to raise the scientific level of medical training; to produce doctors who are scientists practising medicine. This has been an understandable trend given the amazing explosion of knowledge in applied physiology, therapeutics and other medical technologies, but it has reinforced the medical model in its compulsion to define clinical entities with single causes. This, in turn, has led to psychiatrists feeling pressures on themselves to obtain equal status with specialties which have a firmer pathological base to their theories, and they have tended to do this by artificially extending the categories of illness. The low prestige of psychiatry among other disciplines has resulted in many doctors still having had only a poor exposure to the challenging nature of this area of medicine and has produced doctors who feel much happier dealing with definite physical illness. There is also a tendency to give patients with emotional disturbance a hard psychiatric label to justify the use of a psychotropic drug.

It is important to remember that in addition to being a professional, a doctor is human and is likely to have prejudices and problems himself. If he has marital or alcohol problems or is tired and bad-tempered, these are all likely to interfere with the way in which he assesses his patient and handles the consultation. In addition, if religious, financial interest or other values enter into his view of his patients' problems, he may deceive himself that he is being a doctor when in fact he is also being an evangelist or entrepreneur. These personal value perspectives of the doctor are not usually made explicit to patients joining a practice list. Patients may be unaware that they are influencing their management or, if they are aware, they may be incompetent to seek a second opinion.

The Patient

Differences in what is seen as constituting illness can arise in many ways. Different ethnic and social class groups perceive illness in differing terms. The process of decision involved in consulting a doctor depends not only on the way the patient feels his distress, but also on the way in which it is felt and seen by his spouse, family and employers. Over the years of married life, couples come to resemble each other in their degree of neuroticism, and tolerance of abnormal behaviour is likely to occur unless some grossly embarrassing or obviously abnormal event occurs. This is especially the case with elderly patients beginning to dement, where the acknowledgement of the condition by a spouse will mark the beginning of the end of their lives together. On the other hand, with grossly disturbed psychotic episodes of a schizophrenic or manic kind, it is likely to be the family and not the patient who complains. In conditions of full employment and protection of jobs by strong union organization, the disadvantage and even disaster of major illness is minimized. However, these conditions are still not universal. Conscientious or exploited employees may well deny their difficulties until a very late stage, for fear of the consequences.

Sick Role and Scapegoating

It is not possible to consider this subject without paying attention to the concepts of the sick role and of scapegoating. In every culture, for a person to be designated as sick imposes certain obligations and rights on him. He is exempt from his working and social responsibilities and instead is sanctioned in his temporary or permanent dependence on family or community for support and succour. These are obviously important social devices for caring for the sick and ensuring a quick recovery where this is possible, but such a role has attractions to people who have difficulty in sustaining an adult relationship with the world, with its ensuing obligations. In the past people who were suspected of illicitly assuming the sick role have tended to be labelled as malingerers or hysterics, but these can be dangerous labels in their implication of the absence of a problem lying in the legitimate area of medical practice. Eliot Slater (1965) described a group of patients who had been given a diagnosis of hysteria whom he had followed up at the Queen's Square Hospital for Neurological Diseases. In this group of 85 patients, followed up for an average of nine years, 12 died, 14 became totally and 16 partially disabled and only 43 remained independent. The further diagnoses included varying malignancies and multiple sclerosis. It seems that if a diagnosis of hysteria is to be made, it should always be qualified by a second diagnosis, whether of personality disorder or whatever.

More recently, Kendall (1974) has suggested a classification of illness behaviour dependent on the amount of recognized and unrecognized disease present and the advantages to the individual of the invalid role, or illness behaviour which may be motivated by a fear of disease or death. Certainly the attendance of large numbers of men for sickness certification on Monday mornings should prompt much wider questions about the meaning of the attendance. If we are really concerned about the total health of our patients, then to accept facile explanations about their earning sufficient 'on the sick', while ignoring the incidence of undetected alcoholism or of alienation from their work, is to confuse inborn prejudice with professional assessment. To arrive at a full understanding of the meaning of the consultation, we must know why this person has attended now.

In the same way that a person who is severely disordered may fail to attend his doctor, it is not uncommon to find a situation where one must ask whether the one attending is the real patient. The concept of scapegoating is one that has been proposed in the USA as an explanation of schizophrenia. This is based on the assumption that it is family communication patterns that are at fault, and that when the family can no longer function with the disturbance, one member may be singled out by the rest and labelled as the deviant or sick one. While there is no evidence to support this explanation of schizophrenia, it is undoubtedly true that some parents have a tendency to see adolescent behaviour which they cannot accept in terms of illness, and the family doctor may be under pressure to label one person as ill when a family interview might be more appropriate.

A key to understanding the relationship of a patient to his presenting complaint is an understanding of his premorbid personality. The family doctor is in a prime position to have acquired this understanding of his patients over the years, but unfortunately concepts of personality tend to be confused and of a snapshot rather than a dynamic kind. This may lead to confusing premorbid personality with sickness.

Processes and Developments

The German descriptive psychiatrists stressed the importance of distinguishing between psychiatric processes and what are essentially developments of the existing personality. Attempts were then made to relate body build to personality type and, by implication, to the sort of reactions people show when they decompensate. Kretschmer (1936) suggested that pyknic people tended to be cyclothymic and were more liable to manic–depressive psychoses, while leptosomatic people were more likely to become schizophrenic. This view was developed by Schneider (1923) who applied the concept of statistical abnormality to a variety of descriptive personality types. The dangers of this approach are obvious in that it is likely to encourage a view of personality as fixed and to encourage a tendency to classify according to a predominant personality trait rather than taking into account developmental, interpersonal and environmental aspects of the way people behave and feel. Schneider's basic approach continues to this day (Table 1), and has been extended to derive concepts of psychopathy and sociopathy. In this country the preoccupation with

Table 1. A classification of personality deviations and neurotic reactions (Slater 1965).

 1. Depressive reactions
 2. Neurasthenic reactions
 3. Anxiety reaction
 4. Hysterical reaction
 5. Depersonalization reaction
 6. Anorexia nervosa
 7. Obsessional states
 8. Irritability
 9. Hypochondriasis
10. Paranoid reaction
11. Unstable drifter
12. The cold and emotionally callous
13. Sexual perversion

intelligence and a tendency to ignore other aspects of personality probably reflect our cultural values.

The influences of psychoanalytic and psychodynamic theories, together with ideas about the fluid nature of personality development, have led to criticism of attempts to categorize personality in this way. In particular, Walton and Presley (1973) have suggested that it is much more useful to try to look at the dimensions of personality. This is especially the case in general practice where we are dealing with such a wide range of 'normal' behaviour and experience and where the extreme deviant is comparatively rare.

Sullivan et al. (1957) in the USA developed a system of describing personality based on the idea of a core structure and developmental stages of personality integration. This scheme was principally developed for use with offenders, but as a framework it is useful in many settings. They propose that individual personality has a tendency to integrate and stabilize, providing a core for further growth and that this is exposed when under stress. However, the core may be modified by further experience and itself provides the basis for further experience by affecting the way the person approaches the world. They define seven integration levels ranging from a schizoid level, where it is not possible for the individual to lead a separate existence, to a level where the person is flexible and able to initiate and cope with change in an adaptive way. At each level there is a crucial interpersonal problem to be solved (Table 2). Most adults probably function between levels 5 and 6.

More recently, Eric Berne's concepts, which have been developed into the theory of transactional analysis, have had a wide influence on the way in which

Table 2. Levels of integration of personality (Sullivan et al. 1957).

Level	Characteristics
One	a) Confusion between self and non-self; a tendency to generalized anxiety reactions.
	b) Dependent on the environment but has no understanding of how it operates and may be overwhelmed by own primitive feelings.
	c) Magical thinking, powerful primitive fantasies and inability to postpone gratification.
	d) Inability to understand a different point of view.
	e) Bound to be at odds with society (adults found in mental hospitals, on skid row, etc.
Two	a) Awareness of self and non-self; problem of controlling the world around him; time and space seen as a barrier to gratification.
	b) People seen as a means to an end and in terms of his own needs.
	c) Expects the world to be composed of givers and may operate in a fairly organized way as long as this is true. If this is not true, he may express anger or may suppress his anger and leave the scene with smouldering resentment (go through life feeling misunderstood).
	d) Liable to impulsive aggression.
Three	a) Perception of rules: problem is their integration.
	b) Rules seem to be black and white; assumption being that if no rule is stated, there is no restriction on behaviour.
	c) Tends to test limits.
	d) Understands other behaviour as a reflection of his own and looks for final absolute rules.
	e) No internal guilt but protestations of it.
	f) Types include the conman who assumes that each person will try to manipulate the rules and therefore he trusts nobody and has no long-term relationships; the conformist who plays by society's rules and becomes anxious under circumstances which force him to acknowledge that he is unable to win friends.
	g) Any delinquent behaviour takes the form of 'I didn't see the sign'.
Four	a) Integration of conflict: coming to terms with other people's influence.
	b) Having accepted that it is impossible to control the world completely, he is faced with the problem of being a small part of the total.
	c) Becomes aware of powerful others and of roles.
	d) Begins to select and play roles (identifying with desired figures). He may be a petty tyrant at home or at work and tends to feel tense, suspicious and bewildered.
	e) Reacts to stress in an exaggerated fashion.
Five	a) Problem: differentiation of appropriate roles.
	b) Sees continuity in his own and others' lives, and sees the relationship between his responses in the past, present and future.
	c) Can feel comfortable in his different roles, and shows an appreciation for others and an understanding of what they do and feel.
	d) Begins to see others as complex, flexible people who cannot be dealt with on the basis of a few, simple rule of thumb procedures.
	e) Can empathize with others' happiness; can enjoy people, be stimulated by them and respond to them.

contd

Table 2. (contd)

Level	Characteristics
	f) Can begin to tolerate change and ambiguity in self and others, but may still worry 'who is the real me?'.
Six	a) Problem: distinguishing role from self.
	b) Can distinguish between role and self and may carry out a role without becoming it.
	c) Sees others as enduring because he knows that a person is more than his various roles and shifting behaviour.
	d) Establishes longstanding relationships and goals.
	e) May experience situational anxieties about the welfare of self and others.
Seven	a) Problem: integration of relativity and change.
	b) Unusual to reach this level. No longer seeks absolute realities but sees a variety of ways of living and coping which are equally valid.
	c) Capacity for dealing with people at different levels to himself.

interpersonal behaviour is seen (Berne 1964). Berne's model is essentially a simple one in which he sees people as having Parent, Adult and Child roles. These roles are not strictly related to our chronological age, but instead define operational positions that we may use throughout our lives. It may be appropriate to adopt the child role when we are sick or old, and for others to relate to us at those times as parents, but in general the assumption is that during adolescence the child is progressively accorded adult roles and responsibilities and that others will relate to him on an adult–adult level.

It can be seen from this account that personality and illness are multidimensional. These models each have something to contribute to our understanding of what happens when the doctor and patient meet in consultation.

The Doctor–Patient Relationship

The components of illness and personality, of role and expectation, lead to the conclusion that the doctor–patient relationship is most complex. Certainly the consultation is greater than the sum of its parts.

Both parties bring with them different maturity levels, expectations and cultural values. While the doctor may wish to see the consultation as a straight technical transaction, it very rarely is. In particular, there is likely to be a confusion about the nature of the differing roles that each party requires in dealing with the other. The traditional doctor–patient relationship, dealing as it does with one person's supposed superior knowledge and skill and the other's ignorance and distress, has tended to be one in which the doctor relates to the patient as a parent to a child. In modern times with changed expectations, levels of education and awareness, the patient increasingly requires to be treated as an equal. In matters of prevention this is not only desirable, but necessary if the doctor is to have any effect. If the patient is kept in the dependent position to have things done to him, he is unlikely to take responsibility for his own actions and health.

Berne's thesis involves the assumption that many interpersonal problems are the result of crossed role communications, such that a patient may be seeking to relate to his doctor on an adult–adult level, but the doctor is used to putting his patients into the child role and relating to them as parent to child. This results in the doctor seeing his patient as an obstreperous (bad) patient and the patient seeing his doctor as a bossy (undesirable) doctor. In this situation, if the participants continue along this path the misunderstanding will remain and the following options are open.

Doctor's Options

1. Continue playing the parent, castigate the patient or have him removed from the list. If he remains on the list, risk poor treatment due to clouded judgement.

2. Give up the parent role and take on the adult role; negotiate with the patient on adult terms, reach an understanding and obtain some insight into your own behaviour.

3. Take up the child role; refuse to face up to the situation, and avoid the patient.

Patient's Options

1. Continue in the adult role and attempt to negotiate on an adult–adult level with the doctor. Change doctors if he will not change his role.

2. Give up the adult role, take up the parent role and have a major confrontation.

3. Give up the adult role, take up the child role, placate the doctor and be a good patient on the doctor's terms.

Assessing the Situation

The doctor's and the patient's assessments of the situation may well differ, with an area in which the doctor sees illness where the patient sees none and the patient sees illness where the doctor sees none. The congruent area will include what might be called 'agreed illness' where the doctor, although not convinced, is prepared to accept the patient in the sick role as part of his strategy, although not having defined any disease entity (Figure 1). This area will include those people where the effect of a placebo is felt to outweigh the effort required to stop prescribing it and those people on psychotropic drugs which have effectively become a placebo, and which the doctor has given up trying to stop. In this case it is important that the doctor acknowledges to himself what he is doing. The category will also include those patients for whom sickness-certification represents an appropriate course of action in view of the various family circumstances.

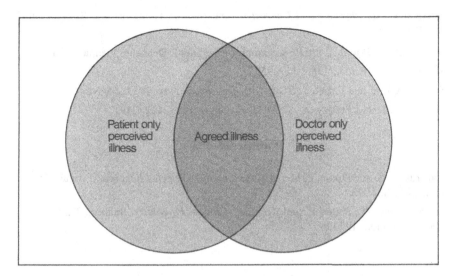

Figure 1. *Perception of illness*

The medical consultation itself consists of an ordered sequence of stages, which have been explored by Byrne and Long (1976). It is salutory to note that in interviews analyzed by Byrne, the occurrence of the 'by the way doctor' phenomenon was associated in a large number of cases with a failure by the doctor to follow information given by the patient, which would have led to the real reason for attendance.

Attendance at the surgery represents for many people the end point of an awareness of malaise, anxiety and self-examination. This is often associated with some regression in their level of functioning and the arousal of primitive, magical expectations. In this respect, western medical practice has been found to differ little from that of native doctors in the Third World. This in itself can be a potent source of therapy as indeed can the communication by the doctor of his empathy with the patient's distress. The doctor has always, in his position, several roles, which are as important as the Pharmacopoeia in the way he uses them. If he can appropriately slip in and out of the role to suit the needs of particular patients on particular occasions, his need for the scientific black magic offered by writing a prescription is likely to be much reduced.

References

Berne, E., *Games People Play*, Penguin, Harmondsworth, 1964.

Byrne, P. S. and Long, B. E. L., *Doctors Talking to Patients*, HMSO, London, 1976.

Kendall, R. E., *A New Look at Hysteria*, Medicine Add On Series, 1972–74, No. **30**, p. 1790.

Kretschmer, E., *Physique and Character*, (2nd edition), Routledge and Kegan Paul, London, 1936.

Schneider, K., *Psychopathic Personalities*, (9th edition), Deutiche, Vienna, 1923.

Slater, E., *Br. Med. J.*, 1965, **1,** 1395.

Sullivan, Grant and Grant, *J. Study Interpers. Proc.*, Nov. 1957, **20,** No. 4.

Walton, H. J. and Presley, A. S., *Br. J. Psychiat.*, 1973, **122,** 259.

Further Reading

Lazarus, R. S. and Opton, E. M. (eds), *Personality—Selected Readings*, Penguin, Harmondsworth, 1972.

Mayer-Gross, W., Slater, E. and Roth, M., *Clinical Psychiatry*, Baillière, Tindall and Cassell, London, 1970.

2. Psychiatric Epidemiology

While the origins of the epidemiological method are firmly rooted in the study of infectious diseases with their largely single causal agents, the discipline has been used widely in answering questions about the distribution and pathogenesis of conditions with multiple causal factors. It is seen as a basic tool in the evaluation and planning of medical services. It is notable that psychiatric disorders, which are such complex phenomena, have been subject to a considerable amount of attention from epidemiologists. This probably reflects the failure of traditional avenues of pathological investigation to produce aetiological answers.

Society and Mental Illness

Men have long been fascinated by the relationship between society and mental illness. As Arthur (1971) has stated, 'only scientific physicians have ever doubted that events in life influence the start of disease'. Pinel was aware of the higher incidence of mental disorder in the single, compared with the married, person (Slater and Roth 1970), and it is commonly supposed that the prevalence of mental disorder is increasing with 'the stress of modern life'. In fact this is a remarkably difficult hypothesis to substantiate. It is in an attempt to test this and similar hypotheses about the effects of other factors, such as age, sex, social class and race on mental illness, that psychiatrists have turned to epidemiology for help.

As Mechanic (1970) has pointed out, the epidemiologist relies on disease as his dependent variable, and this immediately demonstrates the weakness of psychiatric data. Epidemiological investigation assumes that the disease under consideration can be accurately defined and assessed, an aim that is most convincingly achieved when definite pathological findings can be demonstrated and which is least convincing with the subjective phenomena of emotion. Definitions of mental disorder fail to distinguish social values and social risks from pathology; while alcohol and tobacco are harmful and satisfy psychological needs, it is usually only alcohol that attracts a psychiatric label. Similarly, other dangerous activities, such as motorcycling and mountaineering, have been ignored, while experimenting with proscribed drugs has been included in the net. Mechanic points out that the tendency to view the

Irish lower-class drinking pattern and the Negro adolescents' experimentation with narcotics as potentially pathological, but not the equivalent attempts to find kicks and excitement characteristic of the more affluent classes, suggests perhaps some biases inherent in psychiatric epidemiology. He suggests that it might be more useful for the epidemiologist to focus on high-risk behaviour rather than on the concept of psychological disorder as used by psychiatrists. From the viewpoint of general practice, attempts to apply narrow systems of classification, such as the International Classification of Disease, to the common emotional disorders in the community may give misleading results (Shepherd et al. 1966).

The epidemiological approach is used to arrive at reliable measures of the incidence and prevalence of specified disorders. Attempts are then made to relate these rates to differing factors in the composition and way of life in the communities under consideration. Studies have been carried out with hospital populations and in the community through community mental health registers, surveys and by special studies in general practice. Attempts at assessing the changes in the prevalence of mental illness over time are confounded by such administrative changes as the construction of the mental hospitals in the last century, the development of outpatient psychiatry, improved access to psychiatry as a result of the extension of medical care, the development of effective pharmacological treatments and changes in public attitudes towards mental illness, all of which have effects on the demands for care. To what extent there are any changes in needs remains problematical.

There is some evidence to suggest that immigrants are more likely to develop mental illness than fellow countrymen who remain at home, but whether this is a result of the tendency of unstable people to migrate is uncertain. Similarly, schizophrenics of lower social class are over-represented in the central twilight areas of towns. The issue as to whether this is the result of migration into these areas by people who are not functioning well or whether adverse social conditions have a causal relationship to schizophrenia continues to be contested. In general it has been found that admissions to psychiatric units are more common among the single, widowed, separated and divorced.

Prevalence Studies

The best-known surveys of prevalence of psychiatric disturbance within communities are those which were carried out in midtown Manhattan (Srole et al. 1962) and Stirling County, Nova Scotia (Leighton 1961). The midtown Manhattan study indicated that 23 per cent of the population suffered from serious psychiatric symptoms, while the Stirling County study found 20 per cent.

The first large-scale British study was on samples of 46 Greater London general practices (Shepherd et al. 1966). Information was obtained on a one-in-eight sample of all patients seen in the practices throughout the year, and psychiatric illness was classified into five main groups of formal psychiatric illness and five subsidiary groups of psychiatric-associated conditions:

Formal psychiatric illnesses:

1. Psychosis (schizophrenia, manic–depressive psychosis, organic psychosis).

2. Mental subnormality.

3. Dementia (deterioration of mental powers in excess of normal ageing process).

4. Neurosis (anxiety state, depressive, hysterical, phobic or asthenic reactions, others).

5. Personality disorder.

Psychiatric-associated conditions:

1. Physical illnesses ⎱ where psychological mechanisms have
2. Physical symptoms ⎰ been important in the development of the condition.

3. Physical illnesses ⎱ which have been elaborated or pro-
4. Physical symptoms ⎰ longed for psychological reasons.

5. Other psychological or social problems.

It was claimed that this system could be used without difficulty by general practitioners and that it did not conflict seriously with their normal diagnostic habits. The consulting rates are shown in Table 3. These do not represent numbers of patients, as some patients had more than one psychiatric diagnosis.

Psychiatric consulting rates were highest for women aged between 25 and 64 years, with significantly lower consulting rates outside this age range. While the men had the same distribution of consulting rates as the women up to the age of 64 years, these rates were only about half those for the women. There was, however, no change in the rate for men after the age of 64 years. The peak age range for new psychiatric illness was 30 to 40 years, but because of increasing chronicity in middle age, older patients had higher prevalence rates. The proportion of chronic cases was found to be 59 per cent of the male cases and 52.2 per cent of the female. Of the new cases, only 3.5 per cent were referred to a psychiatrist, compared with 7.5 per cent of the chronic cases who were under psychiatric supervision. Among males, the married group had a significantly lower rate than either the single or those in the category 'other', while the rates for females did not differ significantly between the different groups. There were no differences in the rates of psychiatric morbidity in different social classes.

Most patients diagnosed as suffering from formal psychiatric illness were classified as neurotic, whereas psychoses accounted for less than five per cent of the total patients. It is when one looks at the diagnoses that the short-comings of classifications based on hospital practice become most apparent.

Table 3. Psychiatric morbidity in 46 general practices. Consulting rates per 1,000 at risk by sex and diagnosis (Shepherd et al. 1966).

Diagnostic group	Male	Female	Both sexes
Psychoses	2.7	8.6	5.9
Mental subnormality	1.6	2.9	2.3
Neurosis	55.7	116.6	88.5
Personality disorder	7.2	4.0	5.5
Formal psychiatric illness	67.2	131.9	102.1
Psychosomatic conditions	24.5	34.5	29.9
Organic illness with psychiatric overlay	13.1	16.6	15.0
Psychosocial problems	4.6	10.0	7.5
Psychiatric-associated conditions	38.6	57.2	48.6
Total psychiatric morbidity	97.9	175.0	139.4
Number of patients at risk	6,783	7,914	14,697

On the one hand, formal psychiatric diagnostic labels could only be given to 68.6 per cent of cases, the remainder being consigned to 'other' categories of psychiatric associated conditions; and on the other hand, 82.8 per cent of those given a formal psychiatric diagnosis were given that of neurosis. This is most unlikely to resemble the highly selected group of patients seen in psychiatric outpatients with well-developed symptom complexes which enable them to be assigned to ICD subgroups.

This same criticism applies to the National Morbidity Survey (Studies on Medical and Population Subjects No. 26) (Table 4), where 29 per cent of male treatment episodes (23 per cent of consultations) and 22 per cent of female treatment episodes (19 per cent of consultations) are lost into 'other' categories (Table 5).

Problem—Orientated Approach

It would seem that forms of classification, such as those used in the National Morbidity Surveys, are of little use for future work in general practice, where epidemiology seeks to elucidate the relationships and course of common conditions. One way of tackling this difficulty is by using a problem-orientated approach to classification, deriving minimal criteria for awarding problem titles. In this way there is no pressure to force cases into unsuitable classifications, but when a patient develops sufficient symptoms of a category in the traditional classification system, it is reasonable to change the problem title to a diagnostic label. This is likely to be both more fruitful and more intellectually satisfying.

In Southampton, Clark has developed a computerized problem-orientated

Table 4. Episode and consultation rates per 1,000 population by sex and diagnosed condition.

Diagnosis	Episodes		Consultation rates	
	Male	Female	Male	Female
Senile and pre-senile dementia	0.5	1.4	1.1	1.3
Organic psychoses	0.5	0.6	1.5	1.8
Schizophrenia	1.5	2.0	5.4	7.3
Affective psychoses	2.8	6.3	9.2	21.1
Paranoid states	0.3	0.6	1.0	1.5
Other and unspecified psychoses	0.2	0.4	0.6	0.9
Anxiety neurosis	22.4	52.6	45.8	98.3
Hysterical neurosis	0.8	2.9	2.0	8.4
Phobic neurosis	0.8	2.2	2.1	5.9
Obsessive–compulsive neurosis	0.4	0.7	1.8	2.7
Depressive neurosis	16.4	54.6	43.9	132.5
Neurasthenia	1.7	3.2	3.0	5.2
Other and unspecified neuroses	0.4	0.9	0.8	1.4
Personality disorders and sexual deviation	1.1	0.8	3.8	2.5
Alcoholism and drug addiction	1.0	0.8	3.3	1.9
Cardiac arrhythmia	0.2	0.4	0.5	1.0
Frigidity	0.3	0.7	0.5	1.2
Physical disorder of presumed psychological origin	13.3	25.5	24.9	47.4
Insomnia	6.5	12.5	9.2	18.0
Enuresis	2.9	2.1	5.0	3.6
Tension headache	2.8	6.8	3.6	9.0
Special symptoms not mentioned elsewhere, transitory, situational and child behaviour disorders	11.6	16.4	15.9	24.3
Mental disorders (not psychotic) associated with physical condition	0.3	0.3	0.3	0.7
Mental retardation	0.4	0.4	1.0	0.6
Total	89.1	195.2	186.2	400.5

Date from *Morbidity Statistics from General Practice* 1970–1971.

record system for use in general practice (Clark and Bowden 1976). Some preliminary data from a practice of 7,500 patients demonstrate the potential of this approach (Table 6). It is possible to define problems to the level of confidence which is clinically justified and to include the important behavioural and social perspectives which are such a fundamental part of general practice. In this case, the problem statement 'Emotional Problems Undefined' accounts for only two per cent of the problem prevalence. In the data presented it must be remembered that one patient may have more than one problem statement and therefore the totals are of problem prevalence and incidence, rather than of

Table 5. 'Other' categories in the National Morbidity Survey.

	Episodes		Consultation rates	
	Male	Female	Male	Female
Other and unspecified psychoses	0.2	0.4	0.6	0.9
Other and unspecified neuroses	0.4	0.9	0.8	1.4
Physical disorder of presumed psychological origin	13.3	25.5	24.9	47.4
Special symptoms not elsewhere mentioned, transitory, situational and child behaviour disorders	11.6	16.4	15.9	24.3
Mental disorders (not psychotic) associated with physical condition	0.3	0.3	0.3	0.7
Total	25.8	43.5	42.5	74.7
Total as a percentage of all psychiatric diagnoses	29	23	23	19

patient prevalence and incidence. These figures are in broad agreement as to an overall prevalence with those of Shepherd et al. (1966) (122 per 1,000 persons at risk), but the inception rate of 133 per annum per 1,000 persons at risk is considerably higher than Shepherd's 52 per 1,000. The practice composition is broadly representative of the city of Southampton. While the figures obtained for many conditions are in keeping with those to be expected from community surveys, one must suspect that the extent of, for example, marital and alcohol problems is grossly under-reported. The whole question of whether it is appropriate to seek these out in one's practice is a vexed one, and a credible view on this must await results of studies of intervention with these problems.

It can be seen that a problem-oriented approach requires that many more problem categories be kept, the advantage being in the increased relevance of these problem categories to general practice use.

References

Arthur, R. J., *An Introduction to Social Psychiatry*, Penguin, Harmondsworth, 1971.

Clark, E. M. and Bowden, A., 'Clinical information and inquiry computer systems (CLINICS)', in *Proceedings MEDCOMP 77 International Congress on Computing in Medicine*, 1976.

Leighton, A. H., *Comparative Epidemiology of Mental Disorders*, Grune and Stratton, New York, 1968.

Mechanic, D., 'Problems and prospects in psychiatric epidemiology' in *An International Symposium of Psychiatric Epidemiology* (E. H. Hare and J. K. Wing, Eds) Nuffield Provincial Hospital Trust and Oxford University Press, Oxford, 1970.

Morbidity Statistics from General Practice, Second National Study 1970–1971, Studies on Medical and Population Subjects, No. 26, HMSO, London.

Table 6. Problem tallies (per 7,500 patients): psychiatric morbidity in general practice using problem orientated records.

Problem title	Prevalence	Incidence to end of:	
		one month (month 6)	year so far (6 months)
Emotional problems undefined	20		8
Enuresis	22	1	14
Marital problems	57	6	30
Anxiety	170	14	87
Agitation	—	1	—
Depression	222	11	90
Phobic–obsessive behaviour	4	—	2
Tension neurosis	68	3	43
Postviral depression	4	1	4
Cancer phobia	2	—	2
Nervous mannerism	2	—	2
Heavy smoker	66	4	60
Unhappy	2	1	2
Pica	1	—	1
Stress reaction	17	3	9
School phobia	7	1	5
Situational reaction	10	—	6
Encopresis	6	—	5
Obsessive–compulsive neurosis	1	—	—
Hysterical aphonia	1	—	3
Cyclic vomiting	4	—	3
Hyperactivity	3	—	1
Nervous breakdown	1	—	1
Agoraphobia	3	—	—
Tension headache	18	3	14
Marital separation	6	—	1
Head banging	17	1	16
Psychotic illness	1	—	1
Schizophrenia	14	—	—
Manic–depressive psychosis	5	—	3
Adult behaviour disorder	3	—	1
Alcoholism	17	—	4
Drug addiction/abuse	48	7	30
Sexual problem	8	1	5
Mental retardation	5	1	4
Paranoia	4	—	1
Attempted suicide	2	—	2
Drug misuse	4	1	3
Personality problem	31	1	7
Heavy drinking	2	1	2
Sleep problem	1	—	2
Loss of libido	3	—	2
Hypochondriasis	1	—	—
Aggressive behaviour	2	—	2
Arteriosclerotic dementia	6	—	1
Bereavement	28	1	21
Total	919	63	497

Shepherd, M., Cooper, B., Brown, A. C. and Kalton, G. W., *Psychiatric Illness in General Practice*, Oxford Medical Publications, Oxford, 1966.

Slater, E. and Roth, M., *Clinical Psychiatry*, Baillière, Tindall and Cassell, London, 1970.

Srole, L., Langer, T. S., Michael, S. T., Opler, M. K. and Rennie, T. A. C., *Mental Health in the Metropolis: The Midtown Manhattan Study* (Vol. 1), McGraw-Hill, Maidenhead, 1962.

3. Anxiety

Anxiety is probably a universal experience and can therefore be regarded as a normal part of the repertoire of human emotional response. However, anxiety states of one sort or another are among the commonest reasons for patients seeing their family doctors. A full assessment of the factors involved is therefore essential to appropriate management.

The Experience of Anxiety

The experience of anxiety ranges from the subjective fears of such things as imminent death and its anticipation, through such subjective somatic experiences as dizziness to objectively quantifiable symptoms, such as diarrhoea and urinary frequency (Table 7). What these factors have in common are modalities of central nervous system connections which interact through the autonomic nervous system and its central connections in the midbrain. Most of

Table 7. The somatic accompaniments of anxiety.

Central nervous system	Tremulousness
	Dizziness
	Headache
	Blurred vision
	Sweating
	Dry mouth
	Insomnia
Psychological	Nightmares
	Poor concentration
	Poor memory
	Depression
Cardiovascular	Palpitations
Gastrointestinal	'Butterflies'
	Diarrhoea
Urogenital	Frequent micturition
	Menstrual symptoms
	Sexual dysfunction
Respiratory	Dyspnoea
	Chest pain

the physical symptoms are the result of the discharge of the sympathetic nervous system. There has been a long-standing controversy as to whether 'the feeling of the bodily changes as they occur is the emotion', or whether the somatic effects and the emotional accompaniments have a common origin in the brain. The consensus view now favours a model in which the endpoint sensation is the complementary experience of centrally felt anxiety and somatic discomfort, which act on and reinforce each other.

From the biological point of view, anxiety represents a state of arousal which prepares the human for a theatening situation—the 'fight and flight' response. Such a response is of great potential value to the individual when he is able to act in an adaptive way. One of the reasons why chronic states of anxiety are so common is that the means of making necessary adaptations in modern life have been lost through a combination of institutional change and individual expectation, such that the individual is unable to make much impression on his life situation even if social institutions encourage this.

The Aetiology of Anxiety

Genetic studies in twins have demonstrated the inheritance of anxiety-prone constitutions. This is not really surprising since physiological parameters tend to be inherited in a normally distributed manner through collections of small genes. What this means in practice is that some people are more likely to develop anxiety states than others, notwithstanding their subsequent life experience. However, it is unusual to find anxious people who do not have other more obviously environmental aspects to their anxiety. The model which has proved to be of most value in understanding the development of anxiety has been that of John Bowlby (1968) with separation. Bowlby showed that there are critical periods in which threats to the integrity of the individual's self-concept and security systems have greater impact than others. The period which Bowlby especially described was that between about nine months and two years of age, when constancy of adult caring seems to be particularly important, and separation is especially likely to lead to disturbance. It seems likely that there are other important developmental points at which anxiety may be produced, and these are likely to be at times of radical change in life situations, (e.g. puberty, leaving home, marriage, loss of a parent, etc.), the so-called developmental crises. The ability to cope with these will depend on previous experience.

In this chapter the four main anxiety syndromes are described.

Specific Monosymptomatic Phobias

It is relatively unusual for a patient to complain of a specific phobia because, generally, these do not interfere with normal everyday living. This group of phobias includes those of thunder and lightning, darkness, heights, water and spiders. People suffering from one of these fears may become terrified at the thought of the situation. Surprisingly, they tend to be otherwise well-adjusted people, except that animal phobias are associated with a high incidence of frigidity.

One such patient was a 20-year-old married woman. During a heatwave when the humidity was rising daily and it seemed that a thunderstorm was imminent, she presented ostensibly with wax in her ears, but her agitation led to further enquiry as to the true reason for consultation. It turned out that she was terrified of lightning!

This sort of phobia responds well to behaviour therapy on the assumption that the phobia is a learned fear response. The most appropriate management is therefore referral to a clinical psychologist who will embark on a course of systematic desensitization, where the patient constructs a hierarchy of the feared situation and then works through it under relaxed conditions, probably with a sedative.

The Agoraphobic Syndrome

The most outstanding feature of agoraphobia is the fear of going into open spaces and of entering shops, buses, restaurants and similar buildings. The condition overlaps and, to all intents and purposes, is to be considered with social phobias, such as the fear of crowded places, of eating or of speaking in public. Because of the severe tension which arises when agoraphobics try to approach their feared situations, they severely restrict their activities and stay where they feel comfortable. Anticipation of the feared situation may be sufficient to induce severe anxiety, with feelings of depersonalization when the surroundings feel strange and unreal. Frustration with themselves may cause them to try to go shopping in town, with a resultant panic attack in the main street, a failure which adds massive reinforcement to the situation.

These patients are often immature, dependent people, whose illness begins suddenly at a time in their lives when they are at a developmental risk point and some threat to their security occurs.

One such patient was a 20-year-old male whose relationship with his girlfriend was turning sour. She insisted on giving him Christmas dinner at her flat and during the day they had a major row and he vomited. Whether the vomiting was psychologically induced or not is unclear, but within two weeks he was unable to enter a public building or restaurant for fear of being sick. Management of his condition consisted initially of exploring with him his feelings about his girlfriend and the reasons for the row. This turned out to be related to his relative immaturity and fear of being tied down, while simultaneously having become dependent on the girl. It undoubtedly helped him to see this, and it was then possible to embark on simple desensitization by putting him on a regular dose of diazepam (Valium), 5 mg q.d.s. and working out with him a protocol for undertaking the feared situations. He was initially barred from trying the most difficult situations. In the first week he had to walk past and look in as many restaurants as he could. The following week he had to go into a restaurant and order a small meal, which he ate successfully, and by the third week he was able to go into a restaurant and eat a full meal.

The family doctor's role in treating disorders of this kind can be crucially important, because patients are likely to present early to him if he is alert and early treatment produces excellent results. Delay in treatment leads to reinforcement of the symptoms and the sort of demoralizing course which leads to patients spending their daytime hours in psychiatric day units. It is often important to be prepared to use fairly high doses of a benzodiazepine. Diazepam 10 mg t.d.s. or q.d.s. is not unreasonable at the beginning of treatment, but the necessity of negotiating a plan with the patient on the understanding that the tablets and the intervention are both an interim crutch cannot be overstressed. These patients readily become dependent on both the doctor and the tablets.

Psychosomatic Syndromes

Given the variety of somatic symptoms which may accompany anxiety, it is not surprising that these may often be produced to the doctor as the presenting symptom. This is an area fraught with danger, because of the tendency to deal in physical terms with an emotional illness and the tendency to ignore physical symptoms in patients with a known history of psychosomatic disorder. The first course leads to a confirmation and reinforcement of the sick role and often considerable expense to the health service. The second course leads to undiagnosed serious illness. The good clinician takes a full history, examines where appropriate and always keeps an open mind.

A 30-year-old estate agent presented with a two-week history of severe headaches. He was on edge all the time and bad-tempered, but denied feeling depressed. He said that the headache was in the back of his head and that his neck stiffened up. Full physical examination was negative, but he consistently denied any emotional problems for five weeks until he had a row with his boss and resigned from his job. At the interview he was tearful and admitted to long-standing tension at work which he found difficult to cope with. He found a new job, the headaches ceased and did not return.

Patients with this sort of presentation are often psychologically very defended. They are unable to admit to themselves or their families when they are in difficulties and they can be very frustrating to treat. Out of this frustration often comes an organic referral, when a re-examination of life goals would be the most appropriate action.

Diffuse Situational Anxiety

The groups discussed so far are fairly straightforward in terms of the ease with which they can be classified and subsequently managed. However, there are many people who present to the doctor with a much more complicated mixture of physical, emotional, work and family problems, and for whom a full understanding of the problem is only likely to unfold with time and with the benefit of detailed past records. These patients have problems of living, and it can be difficult to assess the meaning of an isolated consultation without the longitudinal perspective of family practice care.

One such patient was a 35-year-old married lady with three children who complained of crying and feeling agitated and unhappy. She had no diurnal variation of mood and her sleep and vegetative functions were normal. Her home life was very unhappy, and it was apparent that there were a lot of family problems. The records revealed that the children were being supervised by the social services department because they were regarded as being at risk for non-accidental injury and the patient herself was regularly beaten by the husband.

The management of this sort of problem requires careful attention to the social as well as the psychological factors; good liaison with the social worker involved is mandatory. Again, it is important that medication should not be used as a substitute for more appropriate action, which in a case like this may well be to provide support for the woman in her decision to leave her husband. However, medication has a part to play, albeit as an adjunct to the doctor's therapeutic role, in making it clear that he understands the patient's problems, that he is prepared to offer support either through himself or through the social worker, but that he is not prepared to start her on open-ended medication.

The Role of Medication and Psychotherapy in the Treatment of Anxiety

From the examples described, it can be seen that a clear analysis of individual cases is fundamental to adequate management. While tranquillizers and sedatives have their place in management, they must be regarded as only a part of the total care; listening to patients and clarifying with them the nature of the problem is equally important. It cannot be stressed too much that a plan of management is essential at the outset. This may be modified with time, and it may in fact come to be that of an 'agreed illness', with mutual acceptance of the need for continued prescription of psychotropic drugs. However, unless a critical approach is adopted from the beginning, it is not possible to end prescriptions for many people at a later date when they can well do without them.

As with all prescribing, it is best for the doctor to become familiar with a small number of drugs and to use them widely. In recent years, large numbers of psychotropic drugs have come on to the market, many of them belonging to the benzodiazepine group. There is little to choose between them and the family doctor is well advised to use diazepam (Valium), which is the cheapest and comes in a flexible range of tablet strengths. He can then experiment with different levels of the drug and develop a thorough working knowledge of its potential and a confidence in prescribing high doses when these are indicated.

Some patients suffering from severe acute anxiety may need a stronger preparation. In these cases trifluoperazine (Stelazine) 2 to 5 mg t.d.s. is often of great value; it is a very useful back-up preparation to a selected benzodiazepine.

Conclusion

The explosion of developments in psychotropic drugs has led to much confusion in their prescribing. The cost of prescribing them uncritically is becoming enormous. However, we are now reaching a position where our theoretical understanding of the aetiology of anxiety symptoms can be matched by a hardheaded and realistic approach to management.

Reference

Bowlby, J., *Child Care and the Growth of Love*, Penguin, Harmondsworth, 1968.

4. Depression

The feeling of depression is a normal part of the human emotional response, culturally accepted and accommodated for through ritual in such situations as bereavement. Increasingly, however, patients present to their doctors complaining of anything from sadness to profound depression with the expectation of receiving medical help; as likely as not they will receive a prescription for a tricyclic antidepressant. To what extent is this a rational management? Is it appropriate at all and how can the management be refined?

Classification of Depression

Much confusion surrounds the classification of depression, not only because of the ambiguous labels used to describe it, but also because it almost seems to have passed above the heads of mere mortal doctors on to the plain of statisticians armed with multivariate and cluster analysis. Labels are confusing because they mix descriptive and aetiological classification systems at a time when hypotheses about aetiology can only be tentative. Thus, psychotic depression, which is characterized by a number of biological symptoms such as early morning wakening, psychomotor retardation and perhaps constipation, is also referred to as endogenous depression, implying that the cause is known to be from within. Similarly, neurotic depression, with its pejorative implications about the previous personality and its lack of the more biological features, is also referred to as a reactive depression, implying that the mood is reactive to circumstance (in both directions). It is no wonder that students and doctors alike despair.

In an attempt to clarify the situation, psychiatrists from the Newcastle, Leeds and Maudsley schools have become locked in argument over statistical analyses. The Newcastle school claims to have defined two distinct populations: the endogenous depressives and the reactive depressives. The Leeds and Maudsley schools claim that the data demonstrate a continuum from sadness to psychotic depression. The general practitioner faced with an unhappy housewife needs to be able to come to a rational, speedy formulation to enable him to devise an appropriate remedy. The danger of the debate that has been enjoined is that it fails to provide guidelines, and results in doctors taking either a prescribing or a non-prescribing line. It is mandatory in assessing emotional problems to pay due attention to the environment as well as to the genes, and a balance must be struck between the loading placed on the presence of the biological features of depression and the significant life difficulties which seem to have a direct bearing on the situation and which need tackling.

If three or four of these symptoms are not present, then it is neither fruitful nor helpful to prescribe antidepressant medication, since the net result is to confirm the patient in the sick role with its denial of individual involvement and responsibility or potential scapegoating by the family or significant others. It is likely to lead to longstanding dependency on medication and on the doctor and a poor prognosis compared with an otherwise good prognosis. Management along the lines of permissive use of psychopharmacology is often defended on the grounds of the doctor's limited time, but if the time involved in seeing a patient who has become collusively dependent on the doctor is compared with the extra time taken at one or two initial interviews to define the problem more clearly, this argument begins to look shortsighted.

One must be alert to the key biological featues of depression, since these features will generally be found to respond to treatment with anti-depressant drugs, whether or not counselling is required in addition.

The Biological Symptoms of Depression

The biological symptoms of depression are:

1. Good premorbid personality.
2. Sudden onset for no good reason.
3. Qualitative difference from normal sadness.
4. Retarded psychomotor activity.
5. Early wakening.
6. Ideas of guilt.
7. Nihilistic, paranoid or somatic delusions.

Aetiological Theories of Depression

Genetic studies of twins have been inconclusive in unravelling the exact nature of any inherited predisposition to depression. What they do demonstrate is that, for depressions of the more psychotic type, there is a definite genetic component, but that this is not a straightforward major gene inheritance. The nature of the inheritance could be explained either by major gene inheritance with partial penetrance (about 30 per cent) or by polygenic small gene inheritance (as with height or weight). A diathesis stress model for the appearance of a depressive illness in a particular person would be in keeping with these explanations and it would predict that the stronger the family history, the less the environmental stress required to cause a breakdown.

If an item of behaviour can be shown to have genetic aspects, then it is perti-
nent to ask what is the effect of such behaviour on the species viability. About
eight per cent of men and 16 per cent of women can expect to have a
depressive illness during their lifetime; a prevalence of this order must have
some positive biological value for the genes to be sustained at this level in the
population, unless there is a high rate of mutation.

It has been suggested that psychotic depression has similarities to hibernation in other animals. However, man does not appear to have any of the
equivalent physiological characteristics necessary to ensure survival through
hibernation.

Sir Aubrey Lewis (1934) suggested that depression enables the individual to
withdraw from a noxious situation, to regroup his resources and to emerge to
live another day. Unfortunately, depression affects all aspects of the individual's life and can result in self-destruction, which can hardly have any
adaptive value as far as the individual is concerned.

Studies of animal behaviour have demonstrated the importance of hierarchy
and territory in determining social interaction. The demotion of a high-ranking
male vervet monkey as a result of a challenge by another monkey results in the
scrotum of the loser becoming pale and in the animal behaving in a manner
remarkably similar to a human with psychotic depression (Price 1972).

Other studies have looked at the effects of separation of monkeys from their
mothers and peers, and demonstrated an agitated depressed state often accompanied by apparent searching behaviour (McGinnis 1979).

If psychotic depression has an important genetic component, as it seems to,
then at some point in the neurophysiology of the hypothalamic–limbic system,
it ought to be possible to define aberrations in depressed patients. As a result of
observations on the effect of reserpine and monoamine oxidase inhibitors, the
so-called catecholamine theory of depression stands as the current theory to
explain both the mediating pathways of psychotic depression and the mode of
action of anti-depressant drugs. The assumption is that patients with psychotic
depression have reduced levels of neurotransmitters in the centres of the brain
concerned with mood. These levels of transmitters (dopamine, noradrenaline and
5-hydroxytryptamine) are increased by tricyclic antidepressants, monoamine
oxidase inhibitors and electroconvulsive therapy.

The Treatment of Depression

Counselling

Ivan Illich (1975) has forcefully stated the proposition that we live in an age
which denies the pain of living. Through the pain of the trauma which occurs in
the course of our normal lives comes personal growth and resilience. To
cushion every traumatic event with medication is a questionable blessing, and

for most distressing experiences what is required is not a prescription but a sympathetic and constructive ear. The doctor should be prepared to use this and to see it as a valid alternative to medication. Unfortunately, counselling is one of those skills which it is assumed every doctor possesses, and only recently has any interest been taken in training doctors in much needed counselling skills. The aims of treatment, as defined by Long et al. (1976), are:

1. To define the problem.
2. To generate solutions to the problem.
3. To examine the solutions in a practical way.
4. To support the person in selecting a solution for himself.

When doctors feel more at ease with this approach the logarithmic increase in prescription for psychotropics may begin to level out.

Patients with severe depression should not be approached with a counselling technique until they are feeling better, since further introspection may lead to suicide.

Tricyclic Antidepressants

In a patient with several biological features of depression, and in particular early morning wakening with brooding, depressed thoughts, suicidal ideas or delusional beliefs, tricyclic antidepressants are the drugs of first choice. As with the benzodiazepines, the pharmaceutical manufacturers pursue a line of introducing many new preparations differing only slightly from those already available. It is best to become familiar with one preparation and to stay with it. Amitriptyline hydrochloride sustained release (Lentizol) is probably as good as any of the available preparations and has the advantage of needing to be taken only once daily. A starting dose is 50 mg for most people, but there is an enormous range in the rate of metabolism which results in some people requiring 150 mg as a therapeutic dose, whilst others require only 25 mg. If the diagnosis is confidently made, then it is important to ensure that an adequate dose is given and taken for sufficient time before deciding that the treatment is ineffective. The tricyclics as a group take seven to ten days to achieve a therapeutic effect, and this tends to be marked by the slight side-effects of dryness of the mouth and some difficulty with accommodation. If a therapeutic response is obtained, it is generally wise to continue the medication for four or five months since this seems to be the order of time for which depressions of this sort last.

Monoamine Oxidase Inhibitors

For patients with severe depressive symptoms in whom a tricyclic antidepressant has failed to help, it is often appropriate to try a monoamine oxidase inhibitor (MAOI). These seem to be of particular value in patients where anxiety, especially phobic anxiety, is prominent.

The reluctance of many doctors to use this group of drugs is based on the fear of producing a hypertensive reaction by combination with sympathomimetic amines or with other drugs. Provided due attention is paid to the contraindications and the patient issued with a food warning card, this should not cause undue anxiety, unless the patient is like the student patient who ate half a pound of cheese just to see if the warning was true!

Phenelzine (Nardil) 15 mg t.d.s. is an appropriate start, though some people will require 15 mg only twice daily, whilst others will require it four times daily for a therapeutic response. The response may take a fortnight or even longer to occur.

Electroconvulsive Therapy

When a patient has severe depression which has either not responded to treatment with antidepressant medication or he is felt to be a suicide risk, electroconvulsive therapy (ECT) may be the treatment of choice; in any event it is time for a domiciliary consultation.

Combined Therapy with a Tricyclic Antidepressant and a Monoamine Oxidase Inhibitor

Combined therapy with a tricyclic antidepressant and a monoamine oxidase inhibitor should only be initiated in a hospital setting, in view of the danger of a hypertensive crisis.

The Presentation of Depression in the Community

Given the confusion that exists about the classification of depression and its origins, together with the wide spectrum of possible mood disturbance from sadness to major psychosis, it is not surprising that depressions can present in many forms. It is of particular importance to pay attention to the person's previous personality and known coping ability, as well as to any family history of depressive illness, in assessing the significance of current life events in causing the depression.

Case History 1—Neurotic Depression

A 21-year-old female clerical worker with a previously unremarkable problem list presented with a two-month history of anorexia and weight loss. She seemed unhappy and withdrawn. After some initial reluctance she divulged the fact that she was in love with her flatmate, but that this girl had now found herself another lover; in the meantime the two were still sharing a bed. Her mood had none of the characteristics of a psychotic depression, being reactive to circumstances and being without delusions or guilt feelings. Nevertheless, she was profoundly unhappy. She was unable to go to sleep, but once asleep she was inclined to oversleep in the morning.

The formulation was that this was a reactive depression in a homosexual girl, her sexual orientation seeming to be quite firmly established.

Management consisted of:

1. Listening sympathetically and helping the patient to clarify the situation for herself.

2. Prescribing a hypnotic (flurazepam (Dalmane) 30 mg at night) for an agreed short period (two weeks).

She was seen on seven occasions over a two-month period, by which time the relationship had been severed and she was dealing adequately with her readjustment. When seen six months later she was completely well.

Case History 2—Psychotic Depression Related To Bereavement

A 42-year-old married woman who had recently lost three relations, including her mother, complained of feeling very tense and irritable, of worrying about everything and being unable to relax. She was having disturbed nights and waking early, feeling depressed. She had lost interest in sex, for which she felt guilty about depriving her husband.

The formulation was one of psychotic depression in a recently bereaved woman of good personality, and management consisted of prescribing a sustained release tricyclic antidepressant 50 mg at night. She made a good response, but subsequently decided to stop the medication as she was feeling so well, and relapsed. Restarting the medication produced a good response, and she remained well when treatment was discontinued after six months.

Case History 3—Personality Disorder, Neurotic Depression and Suicide

A 24-year-old unskilled man, with a history of abusing LSD and cannabis and beating his wife, complained of feeling aimless and depressed because his wife had left him. He demanded Mandrax, saying that if it were not prescribed, he would obtain it illegally. He had no features of psychotic depression.

The formulation was that he was an anxious, unhappy man who had few resources to deal with his situation.

Management was aimed at:

1. Reducing his tension by prescribing diazepam (Valium) 5 mg q.d.s. and nitrazepam (Mogadon) 10 mg at night.
2. Supporting him in coming to terms with his situation.

Over the next few weeks he repeatedly took overdoses of hypnotics and returned to smoking cannabis. He refused admission to hospital on a voluntary basis and, despite lengthy appointments several times a week, he eventually drove into the country and gassed himself with his car exhaust.

Case History 4—Phobic Anxiety and Depression

A 50-year-old publican with a history of chronic anxiety and depression was seen at home on Christmas Eve, when he was complaining of epigastric pain. On challenging him, he admitted to heavy drinking and his wife said he would drink anything he could lay his hands on. Immediate treatment was aimed at relieving his alcoholic gastritis and consisted of:

1. Abstention.
2. Antacids.
3. Diazepam (Valium) 5 mg q.d.s. as a controlled substitute for alcohol.

He was seen a week later and assessed more fully. It transpired that he had suffered from phobic anxiety since being torpedoed on several occasions during the War. For many years he had been unable to leave the pub, and for the previous two months he had become increasingly depressed following the deaths of two of his customers who were close friends. He had resorted increasingly to alcohol for solace. His symptoms were mainly those of weeping for no reason and feeling tense and nauseous in the mornings.

It was felt that this was atypical depression in a man with longstanding phobic anxiety and a tendency to respond to stress by using alcohol.

Treatment consisted of phenelzine (Nardil) 15 mg t.d.s., which had an excellent response after a variety of benzodiazepines and a full trial of a tricyclic had had no effect.

Case History 5—Personality Disorder, Obesity and Masked Depression

A 25-year-old obese mother complained of pain in her knees and ankles. Physical examination was negative apart from the obesity, but the patient was weepy at interview and enquiry revealed that depression was her normal mood with initial insomnia and early morning wakening. She was not an easy person to get on with and previous encounters with doctors had tended to be battles about her weight which she seemed to regard as her doctor's fault or else that of her five-year-old daughter, who she had quite actively rejected.

A diagnosis of masked depression was made and treatment begun with amitriptyline sustained release. She showed no response to a dose of 50 mg at night, but when this was increased to 100 mg, she began to look and feel much better. She said she had not felt so well in six years. With this response it was then possible to begin to look at the reasons for her antagonism towards her daughter.

Discussion

Depression is a diffuse phenomenon and the cases described illustrate a fair cross-section of the sort of problems met with in general practice. With one exception, the outcome was satisfactory. That exception raises the question of how far is it appropriate to strive in the community and whether the patient should have been admitted to hospital on an order? This is a vexed question and one without a clear answer, for the hospital would not have provided anything that he needed that was not available in the community, except a place of safety.

Suicide in the depressed patient is an ever present threat and one not to be taken lightly. Equally it is always important to ascertain of depressed patients whether they have contemplated suicide. Some doctors fear that this will put the idea in the patient's head, but if it is already there, the doctor needs to know.

With a clear formulation and a rational approach to treatment, the management of depression in general practice can be very rewarding.

References

Illich, I., *Medical Nemesis—The Expropriation of Health*, Marion Boyars, London, 1975.

Lewis, A. J., *Ment. Sci.,* 1934, **80,** 277.

Long, B. E., Harris, C. M. and Byrne, P. S., *Med. Educ.*, 1976, **10,** 198.

McGinnis, L. M., *J. Child Psychol. Psychiatr.*, 1979, **20,** 15.

Price, J. S., *Int. J. Ment. Health*, 1972, **1,** 124.

Further Reading

Kellett, J. M., *Lancet*, 1973, **i,** 860.

Sargant, W. and Slater, E., *An Introduction to Physical Methods of Treatment in Psychiatry*, Churchill Livingstone, Edinburgh and London, 1972.

Smythies, J. R., Coppen, A. and Kreitman, N., *Biological Psychiatry,* William Heinemann Medical Books, London, 1968.

5. Schizophrenia

Schizophrenia remains the great enigma of psychiatry. To the layman the condition is synonymous with madness; to the psychiatrist it is likely to prove a major challenge both in diagnosis and in management. The large numbers of chronic schizophrenics still in mental hospitals are just testimony. Yet eminent doctors and philosophers have claimed that the whole thing is a myth, a fantasy created by a medical system of labelling that must seek to reduce all behavioural and emotional deviation to the state of a physiological disease.

Most older doctors had little training in psychiatry as students, though hopefully this seems to be changing. As the policy of community care for the mentally ill proceeds, it is becoming apparent that more than a nodding acquaintance with this most awe-inspiring of conditions is becoming a prerequisite of good practice.

The Diagnosis

The word 'schizophrenia' was first used by Bleuler in 1911, when he applied it to a wide range of disorders found in chronic mental hospital patients. His use of the word in a wide sense has influenced the practice of Swiss and American psychiatry to the present day, so that 'American schizophrenia' ranges from apparently minor personality disorders with a range of emotional reactions, through to the major deterioration of personality that is recognized as schizophrenia by British psychiatrists.

From the British psychiatrist's point of view the symptoms that are present interfere with the patient's thinking, emotions and drive. Patients developing schizophrenia often withdraw from social contact, become sullen, morose and suspicious and spend more and more time engaged in their own thoughts. These may include a variety of abnormal ideas concerning the world about them and the people with whom they are living. They may develop intense feelings of persecution and experience hallucinations, especially in the form of voices commenting on their behaviour and thoughts. The patient's speech is likely to reflect his thought disturbance and will itself become disturbed and illogical, full of outlandish ideas that do not quite relate to each other. It can be extremely difficult to take a history or to obtain a straight answer to a question. An important feature of schizophrenia is that by and large patients are fully orientated for time and place, although this may not be true if they are in a state of excitement. Disorientation usually has an organic cause.

The emotions are often disturbed and, although the commonest disturbance is a blunting of affect, the emotional response may be totally out of keeping with the situation in which the patient finds himself.

First-Rank Symptoms

Because of the wide range of symptoms that occur, attempts have been made from time to time to define a central group of symptoms that could be regarded as having diagnostic significance. Schneider's grouping of so-called first-rank symptoms has come to be seen as a useful guide (Schneider 1959):

1. Disturbances of thought, including the experience of thoughts being put into one's mind (thought insertion), of thoughts being taken out of one's mind (thought withdrawal), and of one's thoughts being known to others (thought broadcasting).

2. Passivity feelings are feelings that one's body, thoughts and actions are under somebody else's control.

3. Auditory hallucinations may take the form of a running commentary on the patient's actions and thoughts and often occur in the third person. These are accepted by the patient as real perceptions, but occur in the absence of any sensory stimuli; they can be neither voluntarily brought into consciousness nor dismissed from it.

4. Primary delusions are fixed erroneous beliefs which have arisen from normal and irrelevant experiences. Fish (1971) gives the example of an Englishman who was standing at a bar with his brother-in-law. The brother-in-law offered him a biscuit from the counter and said, 'Have one of these. They are salty'. Immediately the patient realized that his brother-in-law was accusing him of being a homosexual and was organizing a gang to spy on him.

Schneider's first-rank symptoms are useful because they provide a reference point in clinical situations that are often perplexing. From the general practitioner's point of view an awareness of these symptom areas, and a high index of suspicion when dealing with patients who seem to be undergoing some change in personality, may well lead to an earlier diagnosis—an outcome of the utmost importance for prognosis.

The Dispute About Schizophrenia and its Aetiology

A large number of European studies have reached the conclusion that the prevalence of schizophrenia is around one to two per cent of the population. Thus for a condition with a high morbidity and chronic course it can be seen that schizophrenia is a major public health problem. A general practitioner with 3,000 patients can expect to have between 10 and 20 schizophrenics on his list. The main group at risk for schizophrenia is young adults, although women tend to develop it later than men. This is likely to be the reason why the fertility of female schizophrenics is greater than that of the males, since many women have already had children before their breakdown. In contrast, the men are often unmarried and poorly socialized before their breakdown.

In the past, as patients became known to be ill they were admitted to mental hospitals, where as likely as not, they would stay for the remainder of their lives. With the advent of effective treatments in the form of phenothiazine tranquillizers and especially the depot preparations, it has been possible to adopt radical strategies of care.

Early studies among native New Zealanders and the Bantu in South Africa have been cited as evidence for schizophrenia being a universal condition (Torrey 1973), but this claim has recently been contested on the grounds of poor methodology and the unreliable nature of the diagnoses made. Tropical diseases, such as trypanosomiasis, can cause an illness indistinguishable from schizophrenia. Proponents of social theories of schizophrenia claim that the cultures studied had already been contaminated by contact with western ways.

The opponents of the concept of schizophrenia as an illness draw a great deal of support from sociologists and to a lesser extent from non-clinical psychologists and workers in communications theory. Until recently, although there has been an almost universal dismissal (among psychiatrists) of the idea of social aetiologies for schizophrenia, there has been no cogent critical reply to the antipsychiatrists (however, see Roth 1976).

Those who attract the label of antipsychiatrists include R. D. Laing, David Cooper, Aaron Esterson, Erving Goffman and Thomas Szasz. They hold differing positions in an essentially similar proposition, which draws on the existential philosopies of Heidegger, Kierkegaard and Sartre, the communications theories of Bateson and the game model of human behaviour as expounded by Eric Berne. All these theories share the belief that schizophrenia is caused by abnormal interpersonal relationships and that therefore the rational approach to treatment involves changing these relationships. While there is evidence to show that the course of the illness is influenced by tensions in interpersonal relationships, there is no evidence at all to support the contention that such tensions can be of aetiological importance. The suggestion that they might can only cause further distress to the relatives and friends of the patient.

On the other hand, genetic studies of twins have lent support to two models of genetic inheritance. The first is a polygenic model involving the production of schizophrenia by a threshold effect and the second is that of a single autosomal gene with the appearance of the condition in all homozygotes and a quarter of heterozygotes (Slater and Cowie 1971).

There is no reason why both these methods of inheritance should not be involved. A great deal of research has been carried out on the assumption that some abnormality of neurosynaptic transmission must be present in these patients. So far the results have not been very fruitful. Some people do seem to be predisposed to develop a schizophrenic illness under certain conditions such as childbirth, chronic epilepsy and following head injury, particularly when the midbrain is involved. The relationship to the use of hallucinatory drugs is uncertain, but prolonged sleep deprivation seems to precipitate the illness in some susceptible individuals.

Management

Prompt and effective management is of the utmost importance. While there is little doubt that the pattern of the breakdown and the patient's premorbid personality have a major effect on the outcome (Table 8), there is also little doubt

Table 8. Prognosticators in schizophrenia.

Good	Bad
Acute onset	Protracted onset
Known precipitating cause	No known precipitating cause
Preservation of emotional response	Blunting of emotions
No family history of schizophrenia	Family history of schizophrenia
Normal socialization and previous personality	Poor social development
Early effective treatment	Delayed treatment

that the longer the disturbed experiences persist the greater the damage done to the personality.

Problems in Initiating Therapy

One of the difficulties in management is that where there is an insidious onset, there is a tendency to explain away the symptoms as being accounted for by the patient's personality. The patients may come from families with more than the usual measure of eccentricity and tolerance of abnormal behaviour and thinking, and it is often only after the behaviour begins to affect other people that help is sought. The ascertainment of early decompensation and its effective treatment can result in a remarkably good prognosis.

A problem which often baffles experienced psychiatrists occurs when the clinical presentation involves a mixture of psychotic thought disorder and mood disturbance. Sometimes these patients are labelled as having a 'schizo-affective' disorder which allows for diagnostic fence-sitting until the picture clears. In general terms an illness is likely to prove to be an affective disorder (depression and/or mania) if there has been a primary disturbance of mood. It is quite common for schizophrenics to have a secondary depressive disturbance of mood in response to their illness, and sometimes the fragmented and flighty thoughts can make the distinction from mania very difficult. Often, if asked directly, a schizophrenic patient will admit to having had a sense of persisting unease for several days before the breakdown. This 'delusional mood' may culminate in a primary delusional experience. Similarly, if directly asked, patients will often say they have been sleeping badly with frequent vivid dreams.

Such is the importance of a full baseline assessment that in normal circumstances an apparently incipient schizophrenic breakdown makes a consultant opinion mandatory. However, this is frequently not possible, either because the patient refuses to see somebody, or because at an early stage he may not seem poorly enough to merit a domiciliary consultation or admission under section. The general practitioner is then left with a difficult management decision—should he or should he not start treatment with a major tranquillizer? The answer is likely to be 'yes', since controlling the symptoms takes priority. A detailed record of examples of the patient's appearance, behaviour and actual talk at this time will become invaluable when a psychiatrist comes to review the situation later.

Drug Therapy

Of the major tranquillizers available, chlorpromazine (Largactil) is probably the most widely used preparation, and the range of doses which can be given means that this is a flexible preparation. A dose of chlorpromazine 100 mg two or three times a day by intramuscular injection is usually sufficient to damp down the symptoms, although hospitalized patients sometimes require up to 1 g daily. Extrapyramidal reactions to the drug are quite common but difficult to predict, as they depend in part on idiosyncrasy rather than being a dose-dependent effect. Therefore it is not necessary for patients to be prescribed antiparkinsonian preparations automatically; instead it is better to wait and see whether symptoms develop.

In most cases new schizophrenic patients will be admitted to hospital for assessment. After diagnosis and stabilization, usually with a major tranquillizer (although sometimes if the patient is in a state of stupor or excitement, ECT will be used), it then becomes necessary to devise a long-term management strategy.

Most patients will never be the same again; they will seem to have lost some of their drive and their emotional responsiveness; they often need to take a less taxing job, and their rehabilitation is an important part of management. They will most likely spend some months attending hospital as day patients and later attending a day-centre or an industrial training unit. A social worker who may be attached to the psychiatric unit from the Social Services Department will offer support to the patient in making decisions about his future work and domestic arrangements; sheltered living as well as sheltered work may be necessary. Of fundamental importance is the support and explanation needed by the family and relatives; severe guilt is often intimately mixed with total bewilderment about what has happened.

As the patient settles, his medication may be changed to a more stimulant oral tranquillizer (such as trifluoperazine (Stelazine) 2 to 30 mg daily) or to one of the long-acting depot tranquillizers (Table 9). The latter have the advantage

Table 9. Drug treatment in schizophrenia.

Preparation	Dose	Side effects
Chlorpromazine (Largactil) oral or i.m.	100–1,000 mg daily	Extrapyramidal symptoms Hypertension Skin rashes Photosensitivity
Trifluoperazine (Stelazine) oral or i.m.	2–30 mg daily	Extrapyramidal symptoms (quite frequent) Blood dyscrasias
Pimozide (Orap) oral	2–4 mg increasing to 10 mg as a maximum dose	Skin rashes Extrapyramidal symptoms Possibly glycosuria
Flupenthixol decanoate (Depixol) oral or long-acting injection	Orally 3–18 mg i.m. 20–40 mg by deep i.m. injection every two to four weeks	Extrapyramidal symptoms Possible reactions with MAOI group Possible galactorrhoea Possible depression

of needing to be given only once in three or four weeks and patient compliance is therefore much easier to maintain. Increasingly these injections will be given by the community psychiatric nurse or by the health centre nurse where the primary care team is prepared to take over this duty.

Generally, policy is to keep patients on major tranquillizers for 18 months or two years and then, if they are keeping well, to reduce the dose under observation. Certainly a diagnosis of schizophrenia is not necessarily a life sentence of drug therapy. Continuing support is, however, necessary over the years. Increasingly patients will come to see the family doctor as the person to turn to if things begin to go wrong again—there is no inevitability about continuous psychiatric outpatient follow-up. Life crises that normal people can cope with, even conflicts of personality at work or in the club, are the sort of things which schizophrenics seem to find particularly difficult to deal with and which frequently seem to be related to a relapse. Schizophrenics often seem to need to titrate their social interaction, to be able to venture out into relationships just so far as they feel in control.

Case Studies

Case 1—Paranoid Schizophrenia

The patient, a 30-year-old self-employed craftsman, attended the surgery after his wife had been fined for shoplifting. For some months he had been carrying out virtually no work and his wife had been stealing food for the family. He said that he was living in a dream world, that he had lost interest in everything and had little feeling for his wife, that he felt depressed and weepy and was not eating very well. This mood change appeared to be secondary to his general withdrawal from the world, he was not obviously hallucinated but was very difficult to follow in his talk. He was also very suspicious and refused to enter the consulting room while there was a student present.

At this time he was prescribed a small dose of trifluoperazine 2 mg t.d.s. and was seen again at weekly intervals. As a relationship was established and he felt able to talk about himself, the depth of his disturbance became apparent. There was little in his personal history to raise suspicion about his mental health, apart from his brother who had been labelled psychopathic and had a tendency to violence. The patient said that he disliked crowded places because he thought that people were talking about him, that he believed people were trying to get at him and that things people said to him meant other than the actuality of the words. He often felt anxious, anticipating that something was going to happen to him. He firmly believed that strangers in the street were talking about him, but he would not divulge what they said.

The trifluoperazine had some initial calming effect, but as the extent of the symptomatology evolved he was started on flupenthixol decanoate (Depixol) 20 mg i.m. monthly.

There was a prompt remission in his symptoms and a return of his interest in work, but his feelings towards his family remained indifferent. After six months he requested to stop the injections and remained well three months later.

Case 2—Postpartum Schizophrenia

The 23-year-old patient, who was unmarried and came from an appallingly kept home, became unwell 13 days after giving birth to her third child. She had been walking the street at night in her bare feet, but denied that there was anything the matter. However, she said that the family doctor was God/her husband and that the health visitor was her grandmother. She was intensely involved in a series of mannerisms to do with arranging her fingers in patterns in the air and then saying 'It's three o'clock'. She threw her head back repeatedly and her eyes seemed to roll up. She admitted to hearing voices and throughout the consultation she appeared to be listening to them, but she refused to divulge what they said.

She was admitted to hospital where she settled quickly with four ECT treatments and chlorpromazine 250 mg daily. After four weeks she was discharged home and started on flupenthixol decanoate 20 mg i.m. monthly, on which she remained very well after six months. Indeed the health visitor maintained that the patient was coping better than she had ever known her to.

Case 3—Paranoid Schizophrenia

The 35-year-old patient, who was a spinster keeping house for her elderly father, became unwell over the course of a few days. She was convinced that people were trying to poison her food and that this had been going on for nine months. She had stopped doing her housework and was making bizarre movements with her face and hands. She denied being hallucinated, was not clinically depressed and spoke normally and to the point when asked questions. In view of a history of chest trouble, she was given a full physical examination, which was negative and she was biochemically euthyroid. Trifluoperazine 6 mg t.d.s. was prescribed with a remission of her symptoms and she remained at home. Three months later she remained well and was carrying out her household duties.

Case 4—Chronic Paranoid Schizophrenia

The 54-year-old patient, with a 20-year history of paranoid schizophrenia, had held down a supervised job for some years. About once every two or three years he would become unwell with paranoid delusions and auditory hallucinations. On these occasions he was admitted to the psychiatric unit for a few weeks where he soon settled, once away from the stresses of work. In between relapses he was maintained on trifluoperazine 5 mg t.d.s. and pimozide (Orap) 1 mg daily.

This patient had very little in the way of emotional deficit from his first major breakdown and was now reaching an age when he was feeling regret for what he saw as a wasted life. Many of his classmates from school were successful and had their own houses and cars, and he found this hard to accept.

On one occasion after some friction at work, his thoughts began to go haywire again and he spoke of 'interference by ladies and possibly the Queen'. Two weeks off work and the temporary addition of chlorpromazine 75 mg to his medication settled things promptly. On another occasion he fell off his bicycle and was badly shaken. When seen he was obviously not himself, but a few days off work were sufficient for him to settle down again.

Conclusion

Schizophrenia remains a puzzling, common and devastating condition. The advent of effective drug treatment, together with the movement towards community care of all kinds, will mean that family doctors can expect to have much more involvement in the continuing management of schizophrenics. An understanding of the condition and a familiarity with its management can lead to earlier diagnosis, more appropriate treatment and often the avoidance of unnecessary hospital admissions.

References

Bleuler, E., *Dementia Praecox or the Group of Schizophrenias*, International University Press, New York, 1916.

Fish, F., *Clinical Psychopathology*, John Wright, Bristol, 1971.

Roth, M. *Brit. J. Psychiat.*, 1976. **129,** 317.

Schneider, K., *Clinical Psychopathology*, New York, 1959.

Slater, E. and Cowie, V., *The Genetics of Mental Disorders,* Oxford University Press, Oxford, 1971.

Torrey, E. F., *Schizophrenia*, Bulletin No. 7., National Institute of Mental Health, Maryland, 1973.

6. Child Psychiatry

Disorders in children arouse strong reactions. We have all been through childhood and are likely to have a mixture of pleasant and painful memories of the years of our development and dependency. These residual memories must influence the way in which we perceive the present reality of others going through that stage in their development. In addition, many of us are parents and all parents automatically regard themselves as experts on child care; that expertise is bound by culture and time.

Medical Involvement

Historically the interest in psychiatric disorders of childhood grew from medical involvement in mental handicap. In recent years this interest has been manifested by the development of child guidance and child psychiatry teams working closely together with an ever wider view of what constitutes disturbance in children. A survey of prevalence on the Isle of Wight by Rutter et al. (1970) concluded that a minimum of 6.3 per cent of school children had a behaviour disturbance of some sort, if subnormality was excluded. These could be broken down into those with neurotic disorders (36 per cent), antisocial behaviour (32 per cent), mixed disorders (22 per cent), developmental or habit disorders (5 per cent), childhood psychoses (1.5 per cent), hyperkinesis (1.5 per cent) and personality deviations (2 per cent). In addition 2.6 per cent of the total sample were intellectually retarded, and 4 per cent had a delay in reading ability of greater than 28 months.

In a list of 3,000 patients a family doctor would expect to have about 30 disturbed children of school age. Child psychiatry services tend to be at best patchy and at worst inaccessible. Fortunately, many disturbances in children require minimal intervention other than that involved in bringing them into the open for discussion with the parents and social work support, and the family doctor is well placed to provide effective primary care. If he is able to do this himself and relieve pressure on child psychiatrists, there is more chance that when he has a difficult case or one with a neuropsychiatric component, an early assessment will be obtained. The aims of primary care must be to recognize and treat disturbance as early as possible and by so doing to reduce the likelihood of maladjustment and neurosis in adult life.

With children, the fact that development is still taking place and is occurring rapidly, is both a difficulty and an advantage. It is a difficulty in as much as assessment involves a dynamic situation with the longitudinal aspect of growth based on genetic and constitutional factors and the horizontal aspect based on the environment, relationships and communications with others. It is an advantage in that intervention on its own can often serve as a reference point to the child and his parents and as a means of diffusing the developing tensions, enabling all parties to put things into perspective, while development proceeds and nature itself makes yesterday's problem irrelevant. Left alone, deviation at critical developmental stages seems to acquire a momentum of its own and, if this is already the case, specialist help is indicated.

Freudian Theory of Psyche

Sigmund Freud described three phases of childhood development, the pregenital, genital and latency periods (Tables 10 and 11). His model related

Table 10. Stages of development.

Stage	Type	Age
Pregenital	Oral	0 to 18 months
	Anal	18 months to 3.5 years
Genital		3.5 to 6 years
Latency		6 to 10 years

Table 11. Freudian theory of psyche.

Id	Primitive instincts, wishes, desires and impulses (food, sex and death).
Ego	Adaptive control through experience and educating. This serves a homoeostatic function with regard to the environment by evaluating situations and fulfilling needs when they are appropriate.
Superego	Conscience, control of ethics and morals. This is culture-bound and involves internalization of parents' and others' values.

these to essential psychic energy, which he called the libido, and to the concepts of the conscious and subconscious mind.

He regarded the libido as the essential energy which was used throughout the psychic structure and which was affected by interaction with the environment. As the child developed and came into conflict with the world in its need to fulfil its instinctive drives, it developed defence mechanisms to protect the ego.

Freud's model of pregenital, genital and latency periods reflected his preoccupation with the sexual aspects of development, but it pointed the way to the concept of critical developmental phases where deviations were especially likely to occur. The defence mechanisms that Freud described and which were elaborated by others have entered our everyday language and have become concepts which are regularly used by the most extreme opponents of Freudian theory (Table 12).

Table 12. Defence mechanisms.

Compensation	A common concept physiologically, this was emphasized by Adler psychologically, e.g. small stature, aggressive behaviour, poor self-image and body-building (Atlas syndrome).
Displacement	Replacement of one emotional attitude by another, e.g. taking out frustration with work on spouse, or anger with parents and society on property as vandalism.
Identification	This can be an important developmental mechanism of 'modelling' on a valued adult or a defence against painful reality as in aggressive games or fantasy.
Projection	Disowning attitudes of one's own that one dislikes in other people. If lying is subconscious it may be projection.
Rationalization	Self-deception; finding excuse for one's behaviour or feelings.
Reaction formation	Prudes of Victorian era; intolerance of those parts of other people that one has most difficulty with oneself (protesting too much).
Regression	Reverting to an earlier stage of development in the face of difficulty; that is to say, adopting more of a childlike role which tends to elicit parenting and protective behaviour from others. This can be a normal phenomenon in physical illness.
Repression	Exclusion into the subconscious of feelings which cause guilt or shame. This may be accompanied by selective remembering, and repressed feelings and thoughts may occur in dreams, under stress or under the influence of drugs or alcohol.
Sublimation	This 'conservation of energy' approach led to the idea that artistic achievement was the result of repressed instincts. Sublimation may be manifested in the defence of intellectualization.

Internal Objects and Fantasy

Melanie Klein attempted to produce a model which could explain a child's experience in its first year of life and she developed the concepts of internal objects and fantasy (Segal 1973). In her view, unconscious fantasy is the mental expression of instincts which exist from the beginning of life and are object seeking. For each instinctive drive, there is a fantasy equivalent, e.g. for the desire to eat, the equivalent fantasy is of a breast. An infant going to sleep sucking his fingers contentedly, fantasizes that he is actually sucking or incorporating the breast (internalized object). A hungry, raging infant, screaming and kicking, fantasizes that he is attacking and destroying the breast. Fantasy formation is seen as a function of the ego and is involved from birth in dealing with the impact of reality.

In Klein's view, sufficient ego exists at birth to experience anxiety, use defence mechanisms and form primitive object relations in fantasy and reality.

This immature ego is exposed to the immediate conflict between the life instinct and the death instinct and the conflicts of external reality, and deals with this by projecting the death instinct part into the breast which is therefore seen simultaneously as a good and a bad object. When there is a predominance of good experiences over bad experiences, the ego acquires a belief in the prevalence of the ideal object over bad objects and of the predominance of its own life instinct over its own death instinct. In pathological development, reality is felt as a persecution and there is hatred of all experience of reality, external or internal.

Klein's model is best considered as an allegory because it is undoubtedly and inevitably adultomorphic. How can an adult hope to delve into the psychic secrets of a baby? However, it does provide a vivid idea of the way in which an optimistic or pessimistic view of the world may develop at a very early age and throws some light on ambivalence and the close relationship between love and hate.

Developmental Points

The concept of important developmental points is one that was alluded to by Erikson (1959) in his work with North American Indians. He came to the conclusion that there were eight tasks that needed to be successfully accomplished if a child was to develop a healthy personality (Table 13).

Table 13. Growth and crises of the healthy personality.

Tasks			Stage
Trust	vs	Mistrust	First year
Autonomy	vs	Shame and doubt	2 to 3 years
Initiative	vs	Guilt	4 to 5 years
Industry	vs	Inferiority	4 to 5 years
Identity	vs	Indentity diffusion	Adolescence
Intimacy	vs	Self absorption	Adulthood
Generativity	vs	Stagnation	Adulthood
Integrity	vs	Despair	Adulthood

From E. H. Erikson 1959.

This scheme provides a useful framework in which to consider the other parameters of a child's development when the child has a problem. The sort of questions that need to be asked when faced with a child whose emotional development is going awry are: 'Why has this child become ill in this way now?' and 'How does this relate to his stage of development (locomotor, communication, social, sexual and intellectual)?' If we ask these questions, we are usually well on the way to an understanding of the problem and to placing ourselves in a position where we can help.

Disorders of Habit Training

Parents' involvement in training their children to control their vegetative functions in accordance with cultural norms is part of a wider responsibility over such matters as social behaviour and familiarizing the next generation with those other aspects of culture which are now increasingly delegated to the education service. With regard to the specific training involved over eating, elimination and sleep, parental expectations are a product of the parents' own childhood memories including often unresolved taboos and discomforts and the assimilation of cultural traditions and educational ideas.

The child brings to this situation his unique rates of development which may be more or less like those of his parents and which include his constitutionally derived conditioning predisposition. If training occurs within the context of a stable parent-and-child relationship and supporting wider community, then inherent difficulties from both parents and child may pass uneventfully, but once emotional tensions begin to show, they have a tendency to be self-sustaining.

Eating Disorders

Obesity

It has been thought that overeating resulting in obesity may be either a specific response to a stressful event or a general response to adverse home circumstances.

In a large scale community survey in Newcastle upon Tyne, Wilkinson et al. (1977) found the commonest 'at risk' factors to be obesity in a first degree relative, having an elderly mother, being an only child and the absence of one parent. In particular cases, the factors found to be important will range from these identifiable epidemiological areas through to those cultural fads which have led to 'bonny babies' being equated with fat ones. None of these problems is easy to deal with, but they are more likely to be dealt with satisfactorily if they are brought out into the open, than if they are seen in terms of confrontation with mother and child over the extra pounds. In this case the game becomes a masochistic parent (doctor) to child battle, where it seems that the only person interested in losing weight is the doctor. This is a frustrating situation but an important one. If the doctor finds he cannot handle this sort of problem well, it may be best if he involves the social worker or makes a referral.

Anorexia Nervosa

Anorexia nervosa, in the classical sense of hiding and deliberately vomiting food, is usually only found in adolescents and if it occurs in younger children, it is likely to be a sign of serious disturbance requiring specialist help. The occurrence of this disorder in teenagers, particularly in girls, is probably very common and usually self-limiting. This condition is likely to occur in those who feel uncomfortable and confused about their changing body configuration which signifies the passage from dependency to adult life. The changing body form is an inescapable symbol of the sexual nature of adult life and ambivalence on behalf of the child usually reflects that of the parents.

With the milder forms of anorexia nervosa, the most helpful thing that the doctor can do is to acknowledge that he is aware of what is going on and to provide the opportunity for the patient to share her anxieties with him in a trusting relationship. This simple support is all that is needed for most of these patients, but those who are unwilling or unable to talk about their difficulties may well have a much more sinister outcome (indication of their withdrawal from the world and deep-rooted distrust of adult life). These patients require long-term psychotherapy and the prognosis is guarded with quite a high mortality rate.

Disorders of Elimination

In most children's development, there is an optimum time for toilet training when the child is ready and responsive to being trained. The failure of parents to instigate training at this appropriate and critical time may be the result of fastidious or permissive attitudes. The fastidious are especially prone to instigate an early toilet training regimen. They are likely to be rewarded for their efforts by initial success followed by a breakdown of training consequent on deteriorated parent–child relationships or a stressful event, such as the death of a grandparent or the arrival of a baby sister. With a permissive regimen, what is likely to happen is that by the time the parents realize they have been misguided, their friends are becoming intolerant of the child and the child is past the critical time for implementing training.

Constipation and Soiling

Constipation is often part of a general resistance by the child to its mother's demands, and he is likely to be difficult in his behaviour in other areas. The condition is itself self-reinforcing once hard stools become painful to pass and the toilet becomes associated with pain and fear. Undoubtedly the doctor's first task is to provide reassurance and support to the mother while trying to modify her attitude. The very process of talking about defaecation to a doctor is likely to be a desensitizing experience for an anxious mother.

Secondary soiling usually indicates profound disturbance and, unless it is just an occasional manifestation of regression after a family upset or change, will require a specialist opinion. As indicated in our common language, smearing faeces, leaving packages of it in siblings' chests of drawers, etc. is likely to be an expression of considerable anger. This anger is as frightening to the child as it is annoying to the parents. Unless the child is given the opportunity of developing his alternative patterns of communication to enable him to deal more successfully with his feelings, his rejection by the family will further serve to confirm his deviation and his stunted development.

Nocturnal Enuresis

Nocturnal enuresis is one of the commonest childhood problems presented to the family doctor. It causes frustration and potential harm to the parent–child relationship and good management requires a full assessment including urine microscopy and culture.

Enuresis may be primary or secondary. Primary enuresis is more common in boys and there is likely to be a family history. In secondary enuresis, one is much more likely to find marital or other family problems contributing to a breakdown in control. Once a pattern of bed wetting is established, the child's anxiety over the parents' anger effectively inhibits the acquisition of normal habit.

Management

The first objective in management is to support the mother in taking the pressure off the child. Unless a child is developmentally ready with good daytime control and has an expressed wish to be dry, success is unlikely to occur.

There are four main lines of approach for dealing with nocturnal enuresis:

1. Restricting fluids in the evening and lifting the child before the parents go to bed.
2. Star charts.
3. Tricyclic antidepressants.
4. Bell alarm.

The first of these is contested by some who claim that restricted fluid intake results in concentrated urine and an irritable bladder on the one hand, and on the other, that increased bladder capacity is only acquired if the bladder is allowed to be full. Most doctors prefer to take a traditional view on this point.

Star charts depend above all on the child's motivation and rely on the operant conditioning technique of rewarding desired elicited behaviour—one blue star for each dry night and a gold star for each three consecutive dry nights. The transactional part is equally important because the child brings his star chart with him when he sees his doctor, and their relationship is obviously important in supporting the child's motivation.

It is uncertain how tricyclic antidepressants work, but it has been suggested that they lighten sleep and so enable the child to be aware of his full bladder (these children often seem to sleep very deeply). A 5 ml dose of imipramine hydrochloride syrup (Tofranil) (25 mg/5 ml) at bedtime for a 5- to 12-year-old should be continued for six to eight weeks and then withdrawn gradually. This treatment should only be used when it is judged that the child has a sufficiently mature bladder, the medicine being used to support normal development, otherwise there is likely to be a relapse on discontinuing the medicine with further damaging effects on morale. It is undesirable to contemplate keeping a child on long-term tricyclics.

The bell alarm is a time-honoured device for use with older children. A drop of urine completes the circuit, rings the bell and wakes up the child. It is probably best if the health visitor looks after the practice bell alarm and deals directly with the mothers who need to use this.

It cannot be stressed too heavily that these treatment methods are only part of the total management which must include an assessment of the amount of family disturbance. Depending on that assessment, an opportunity to discuss the family problems with the doctor or other member of the team may be more important than physical treatment in the eventual outcome.

Sleep Disturbance

Apparently the constitutional human clock is slightly more than 24 hours, but this is likely to be a normally distributed characteristic. In the small baby, sleep is governed by hunger and its satisfaction. As the child's metabolism matures and he moves on to solid food, so the time between feeds increases and the period of uninterrupted sleep with it. For some fortunate parents, this happens quite early, and some infants of only a few months will sleep right through the night. The range of parental tolerance of disturbed sleep is wide, and what some parents can shrug off causes night calls to the family doctor by others. With both extremes of parental types there is a danger of developing and reinforcing problems.

On the one hand, a child who feels insecure because of his parents intemperate response to its wakefulness is likely to wake all the more, and is especially likely to find itself receiving some form of hypnotic at his parents' request. On the other hand, tolerant parents may unwittingly be reinforcing their child's wakefulness with the reward of a warm cuddle in the middle of the night. This is most likely to happen if there has been a precipitant to the wakefulness, such as the arrival of a new baby, death of a grandparent or a parent's absence for a few days. The doctor must steer a middle path and this can be very difficult. Not only may some parents be ambivalent about seeing their child in the middle of the night and be reluctant to take a firm line, but others who are unable to be tolerant may have problems of self-control that place the child at physical risk. In such cases it may be appropriate to embark on an agreed period of night medication, such as trimeprazine tartrate (Vallergan) syrup.

Nightmares

Nightmares are common and normal in children of all ages and usually follow a frightening experience. Reassuring the parents is usually sufficient treatment. Night terrors are an unusual manifestation in that the child, usually about four or five years old, wakes up screaming with no recollection as to why this should be. Such events are very disturbing to the parents the first time they happen, but are of no consequence and usually do not persist.

Disorders of Emotion

Emotional disorder in children usually takes the form of an anxiety state, often with regression of behaviour or habits, and accompanied by such physical symptoms as abdominal pain or headache. Depression in the sense that we describe depression in adults is unusual, but a child may be felt to be depressed by his withdrawal and apathy, and certainly any behaviour which symbolically represents suicidal behaviour, such as running away from home or taking an overdose of tablets, should be taken seriously. Suicide is extremely rare in children under 16 years but it does occur, usually following a disciplinary crisis.

Children are usually brought to their family doctor for ill-defined physical problems or unacceptable behaviour, rather than for psychic disturbance per se, and the doctor will only include the psychological factors in his assessment if he is aware of them.

There is a general reluctance to prescribe psychotropic medication for children and it is a pity the same cannot be said about adult patients. If a tranquillizer is felt to be needed, a small dose of diazepam (Valium) on a limited basis while the family problems are dealt with is probably the best remedy.

Disorders of Behaviour

The form in which a behaviour disturbance occurs is usually a function of the child's age. The content of the disturbance is much more likely to give clues as to the severity and nature of any causal factors. The usual problems, in approximate chronological order, are those of school discipline, school phobia, truanting, stealing and promiscuity.

One should first ascertain whether the child is doing whatever it is on his own or whether it is a normal activity for his peer group. It has been shown that more than 50 per cent of schoolboys have committed an offence at some time, but less than four per cent of boys are known to the police as offenders. This is not to say that nothing at all should be made of such an occurrence, because it may be that a child in difficulties temporarily seeks solutions through the nefarious activities of his contemporaries, and that later he will go on to develop his own further elaborations when others have outgrown the activity.

Solitary behavioural disturbance is likely to be indicative of much more profound psychological disturbance. Classifications in child psychiatry tend to distinguish between behavioural and emotional disturbance, but with this particular group this may be a mistake, because these children are often profoundly unhappy. The repetitive truculence and conflict with a teacher may be a desperate attempt to establish a relationship through continuous testing out of the teacher's response, based on an experience of repeated rejection by the boy's own father.

Similarly, truanting may represent a response of 'leaving the field' when all hope of finding such a relationship has been given up for lost. Stealing may be a means of obtaining fleeting financial power to buy the affections of peers, and promiscuity serves a similar function, where sex is the currency rather than money. In all cases, an assessment of the family situation is likely to be the greatest help in deciding the appropriate course of action.

School Phobia

Among behavioural disorders, school phobia stands out as a consistent manifestation of psychic distress. In this case the phobia is not of going to school but of leaving home, and it is entirely different from truanting. While with truancy the child leaves home in the morning and returns at night but does not go to school, the phobic child stays at home in his parents' full knowledge. Truants tend to be of poor families and have poor motivation to academic success. School holds little interest for them. The school phobic child is often of above average IQ and enjoys school.

The failure to attend school occurs on a Monday or on the first day back at school after a holiday, when a panic attack, nausea, abdominal pain or headaches provide the reason for failing to attend school. The condition appears to be similar to the agoraphobic group of disorders in adults, and it is often found that other members of the family have separation anxieties, and that the parents are warm and overprotective towards their children. Usually the child is about 11 or 12 years of age and from the developmental point of view is shortly to enter puberty. The significance of this to both parents and child may be partially understood but not made explicit and is consequently feared.

Management consists of providing firm support to the parents in resisting any effort to keep the child off school and discussing with the parents their fears of the child's growing up and becoming autonomous. The child should be seen separately by either the doctor or the social worker, and encouraged to explore his own fears, perhaps through painting or drawing. If anxiety is prominent, as it usually is, a small dose of diazepam (Valium) on waking may be a useful supporting measure.

The decision to refer to a child psychiatrist must depend on an assessment of what this disturbance means to this child at this time. The family doctor must decide whether this is a passing problem in an otherwise well adapted child, or whether this marks a new deviation of possibly enduring significance. If the latter, he must decide whether his own skills at working with parents and children are sufficient to bring the problem out into the open and deal with it as a family problem or whether to refer it now for specialist help. These are difficult questions and ones that are likely to be answered through acquired experience.

Disorders of Intellectual Development

In recent years interest has developed in the idea of a dimension of minimal brain damage in children occurring either at or before birth and associated with such disabilities as perceptual and learning disorders, overactivity and aggression, and inability to communicate and relate to other people. These difficulties may be associated with abnormal EEGs, but the EEG is usually normal and diagnosis depends on a lengthy assessment by an experienced team which includes a child psychiatrist, a psychologist and a teacher.

From time to time the family doctor is asked by a parent to examine and observe a child who is not thought to be developing normally, despite having seemed to be normal at birth and in the early months of life. These children are noticed when they begin to lag behind their peers on some parameter of developmental function, such as locomotor, language, speech or social development. (In most areas there is now a good service providing developmental assessment with easy access, but the general practitioner needs to have some idea when to use this sytem of referral.)

One of the problems of general practice is that one is dealing with an essentially healthy population with whom reassurance on the grounds that most things get better anyway is normally a realistic approach. However, it is noticeable that the parents of autistic children frequently complain that for several years their doctor told them to stop worrying and it would be all right.

Autism

Autism is a curious condition characterized by apparently normal development for the first 18 months or two years of the child's life, but with development subsequently coming to a halt. Autistic children seem to remain apart from the world and to be unaware of what is happening around them. Such children often have an insistent desire for sameness and will become extremely distressed if, for example, a line of bricks they have laid end to end is disturbed or their daily routine is changed. They tend to be cold and lacking in affection with poor speech development and little facial expression, and avoid eye contact with other people. Their behaviour often has a ritualistic and compulsive quality and they may pursue stereotype movements with their bodies, hands or fingers. One of the most distressing facets of this condition can be their temper tantrums and self-destructive behaviour, such as head-banging. Nowadays it is though most likely that the pathological basis for the condition or group of conditions lies at the level of sensory integration.

Treatment for autism is increasingly based on behaviour modification lines in special units with highly trained staff, but the outcome is usually not very good.

Aspects of the Child–Doctor Interview

Relating to children is a gift which not all doctors have. A child is usually seen with his mother who does most of the talking and the child's part in the interview is minimal. If this format is adhered to with emotionally disturbed children, it is likely that an opportunity will be lost for the doctor to influence the course of events by making therapeutic use of the interview, short though it may be.

After the initial consultation, it is reasonable to suggest to the parents that the child should have his own appointment and that he should be seen alone, unless there is some matter which needs to be dealt with jointly. Often it is appropriate for the mother to see the social worker at the same time as the doctor is seeing the child, for then the mother can receive support and explore with the social worker her part of the total problem. Young children particularly, but often adolescents as well, have difficulty exploring their feelings in a direct way, but will readily paint a picture or set up a play scenario in a sandpit in a few minutes, which is an accurate reflection of the way they feel and see the world. These are invaluable diagnostic and therapeutic tools in a short interview. The shared silence that often occurs while the work is in progress is a valued thing in itself, being felt by the child as unpressured personal time given by the doctor to the child—his own personal doctor and his own personal consultation.

By the time this point is reached, several therapeutic phases have also occurred.

1. The identification of a problem by the parents reduces family tension, because it is no longer denied. The action taken in making an appointment is an indication of motivation to sort out things and the child is likely to realize this.

2. The parents taking time off (from work or housework) indicate to the child something about his importance—an importance he may have come to doubt among all the family tension and recrimination.

3. The first interview, by bringing things out into the open, often enables a problem to be seen for what it is—nowhere near as big as it seemed in the charged atmosphere of home. The doctor's acceptance of the problem is an important transaction in that this implies that this is nothing unusual, he is not going to blame anybody, and the thing to do now is to try and sort it out.

For many children having an appointment to themselves will be the only undisturbed time they have had alone with an adult for a long time. This is a strength and a weakness of the consultation—weakness if the doctor or child seeks this as a substitute relationship, which it can never be, a strength if through it the child realizes that the world can be secure, that it is possible to trust an adult (and therefore why not others?) and to resolve problems, and if in the course of the involvement the parent–child relationship can be helped on to an even keel.

It would be inappropriate and unwise to suggest that family doctors should be doing the work of child psychiatrists, but there is a large morbidity and a shortage of psychiatric manpower. Psychiatrists are best used in a consultative and supportive capacity and for referral of difficult or neuropsychiatric problems. Many of the developmental disturbances of children can be effectively helped by common sense, understanding and four to six 15-minute appointments.

References

Erikson, E. H., *Psychol.*, 1959, **1,** 50.

Rutter, M., Tizard, J. and Whitmore, K. (Eds), *Education, Health and Behaviour,* Longman, London, 1970.

Segal, H., *An Introduction to the Work of Melanie Klein*, (M. Masud and R. Khan, Eds), The Hogarth Press and the Institute of Psychoanalysis, London, 1973.

Wilkinson, P. W., Parkin, J. M., Pearlson, J., Philips, P. R. and Sykes, P., *Lancet*, 1977, **i,** 350.

Further Reading

Lazarus, R. S. and Opton, Jr. M., *Personality*, Penguin Educational, Harmondsworth, 1967.

West., D. J., *The Young Offender*, Pelican, Harmondsworth, 1967.

7. Mental Subnormality

The birth of a mentally handicapped child into a family constitutes an accidental crisis in Caplan's terms (1961). It is likely to result in an immediate state of disorganization and, depending upon how the crisis is dealt with, the strengths of the personalities involved and the availability of external supports during the early critical weeks, the family may emerge strengthened or weakened by the experience.

This crisis can be divided into three parts: the initial shock; the value crisis, which involves a refashioning by the parents of their hopes and expectations for their child; and finally, after months or years, the reality crisis in which parents must come to terms with the day to day practical problems.

If parents discover the fact of their abnormal baby before they have had time to form a relationship with him, outright rejection may occur. When the discovery is consequent upon a protracted period of suspicion, it may have a beneficial effect for the parents, especially if they have a chance to discuss their feelings. There has been controversy as to whether parents should be told immediately or whether disclosure should be delayed to enable parents to become attached to their child. In general, parents prefer to be told early, and uncertainty causes distress. However, it is important to realise that telling the parents is only a first step in the continuing management of the handicapped child.

The Change to Community Care

The change in emphasis from institutional to community care has been a marked feature in the management of the subnormal since the war. Twenty-five years ago parents were advised to place their severely subnormal children in an institution at an early age, but this has been shown to have adverse effects on both the affected child and the parents.

Stein and Susser (1960) have shown that the social class and culture of the parents play a large part in determining whether or not children in the borderline subnormal range are designated subnormal and institutionalized. Boys are more frequently designated subnormal and institutionalized than girls. Stein and Susser found that 75 per cent of subjects ascertained educationally subnormal were clinically free of signs of brain damage and that these subjects made significant improvements in IQ with age. These improvements appeared to have been due to cultural factors which had previously retarded intellectual maturation. Children from social classes I and II are rarely to be found in the ascertained subnormal group, but rather as a small group of severely retarded children with brain damage. Stein and Susser postulate that this is an indication of the latent potential of many previously institutionalized borderline patients to benefit from a full educational and cultural experience which might enable them to live in the community.

The present emphasis is on looking at the child in the family context, with the aim of planning services to enable him to grow up in a local community among ordinary people. One reservation about the current trend of making the lifestyle of the mentally handicapped person as near normal as possible is that it may be attaching too much importance to current values and opinions. It may be that some handicapped people would benefit from a less isolated sense of identity than that provided by a twentieth century Western nuclear family.

Effect on Parents

Studies of the effect on parents of caring for a subnormal child have produced equivocal results. Nineteen per cent of the mothers in Holt's 1957 study of 207 families were exhausted by the physical work and emotional stress involved; marriages were said to be strained by parental quarrelling. However, there was no control group, and the frequency of parental quarrelling (six per cent) is probably no different from that expected in a normal population.

Tizard and Grad (1961) compared families with subnormal children living at home with those of comparable children in an institution. They concluded that families with a subnormal child at home were dominated by the 'burden of care'. This conflicted with the findings of Caldwell and Guze (1960), who found no difference between the mothers of institutionalized and non-institutionalized children. Caldwell and Guze concentrated upon the mental health and attitudes of the mothers while Tizard and Grad looked at social functioning.

Farber (1959), using the Farber 'index of mental integration' found that subnormal boys, particularly over the age of nine years, were more disruptive to a marriage than girls.

A survey of children with Down's syndrome in the Oxford region showed an over-representation of children from social classes I and V who were admitted to subnormality hospitals at an early age. It is likely that the value crisis is too great for the class I parents and the reality crisis, in particular the cost of clothes and household decorations, too great for the class V parents.

Holt (1958) looked at the influence of a retarded child on family limitation. He found that 101 of 160 families did not want more children. In 90 of the 101 families this appeared to be due directly to the presence of the retarded child. Thirty of these 90 families had further pregnancies and 39 of the 101 families relied on abstention or trusting to luck as a form of contraception—a sad reflection on the counselling available.

In all studies of subnormals it is difficult to separate physical from mental handicap as they are so often concomitant. This makes it difficult to assess the effect of heavy nursing on parental attitudes. Another major deficit is the lack of objective data because of dependence on information from the mother.

Effect on Siblings

In Holt's 1957 series, 15 per cent of the 430 siblings were said to be adversely affected; these effects fell into the categories of fear of being attacked, resentment of the parents' attention to the handicapped child, shame, and being overburdened with domestic chores.

Other authors have not found any increased incidence of emotional disturbance among the siblings of subnormal children (Caldwell and Guze 1960). The siblings from stable homes showed strong identification with parental attitudes, and it was suggested that if the parents had been able to adjust to the situation and cope with the practical realities, the other children were unlikely to suffer ill effects.

The Extended Family

The stability of a family with a mentally subnormal child is likely to depend partly on its ability to recruit outside assistance. Farber (1959) found that while close contact with the wife's mother was associated with greater marital integration, close contact with the husband's mother was not. There is no information about the attitudes of other first degree relatives to subnormal children.

Conclusions

The management of the mentally subnormal child is a test of both the family and the community. A family with good maternal and emotional resources and kinship ties may be able to cope at home with a child who is not severely handicapped without adverse effect on the child or other family members, and with little recourse to special community resources.

Families less generously endowed or in a state of fragmentation (Susser's dysmorphic families) are likely to make early demands on community resources. These demands have traditionally been met by hospitalization. In the present health service subnormal children of these families are likely to suffer adverse effects wherever they are placed, and it is unlikely to be of benefit to return them to families ill-equipped to provide for their needs.

Skilled and continuing counselling begun at the time of diagnosis is required to identify vulnerable families and to optimize the management of all subnormal children. Management should be based on a wide and flexible range of facilities which care for subnormal children and adults on a day or residential basis. These facilities should take the form of hostel accommodation, family group homes, different levels of sheltered work, and day care and holiday relief for families looking after subnormal people at home.

A frequent consequence of the move away from hospital towards community care is fragmented team care, and the family doctor is ideally placed to coordinate this throughout the patient's life. To do this effectively he must acknowledge the patient's need and be prepared to arrange and participate in multidisciplinary care, with its inevitable meetings.

References

Caldwell, B. N. and Guze, S. B., *Am. J. Ment. Def.*, 1960, **64,** 845.

Caplan, G., *An Approach to Community Mental Health*, Tavistock Publications, London, 1961.

Farber, B., 'The Effects of a Severely Mentally Retarded Child on Family Integration', *Monographs of the Society for Research in Child Development*, 1959, **24,** No. 2.

Holt, K. S., 'The Impact of Mentally Retarded Children on their Families', MD Thesis, Manchester University, 1957.

Holt, K. S., *J. Ment. Def. Res.*, 1958, **2,** 28.

Stein, Z. and Susser, M., *Br. J. Prev. Soc. Med.*, 1960, **14,** 83.

Tizard, J. and Grad, J. C., '*The Mentally Handicapped and their Families*', Maudsley Monographs, No. 7, Oxford University Press, Oxford, 1961.

8. Aspects of Sexuality

Alex Comfort (1967) has speculated that had the anxiety which has been focused on sex been applied instead to food, the General Medical Council would have refuted any suggestion that a prohibited food might be a useful source of protein while the upholders of 'we know what is right' would have devoted much energy to demonstrating the carcinogenic and pimple-producing capacity of the tabooed articles. Their utmost hostility would be reserved for any objective student who threatened to activate their own anxieties by trying to ascertain the facts. Times have changed and death has replaced sex as the unmentionable obscenity. Meanwhile, the permissive 1960s have produced a generation which, if it cannot actually be shown to be more sexually active than its predecessors, has grown up to expect the same attention from its doctors for sexual difficulties as for more conventionally accepted medical disorders. This mantle fits uncomfortably on many doctors who may have been brought up in more modest times, or who expect that in medicine they should be practising only applied therapeutics or surgery.

The acceptance of the family planning role as a legitimate part of general practice has opened the doors to patients with an invitation to see the functional part of their sexual natures as an appropriate area for medical concern. Increasingly, patients refuse to be satisfied by an endocrine or other organic explanation of problems which they feel to be of a more subtle kind, and they are becoming more assertive in their claims for help; this phenomenon is not restricted to either sex.

Probably the commonest response of busy family doctors to the question of dealing with sexual problems is that this is far too time-consuming, and that if the problem is bad enough to require help, then the patient should be referred to a consultant. When family doctors feel that they do have a part to play, they often feel shy and uncomfortable in dealing with patients' intimate feelings, needs and behaviour. It is becoming apparent that the pool of morbidity and of potential demand is enormous and that there is no chance of there ever being adequate specialist services to cope with it. It also seems that early and adequate intervention in sexual difficulties generally carries with it a good prognosis and that most problems, if dealt with at an early stage, require remarkably little time.

The first step for many doctors who wish to develop this aspect of their work is probably some desensitization towards dealing with sexual matters. This may be achieved through attending one of the training courses in psychosexual problems or by reading some of the very useful texts now available (see Further Reading).

The Development of Sexuality

The roots of our sexuality remain obscure. They are likely to include some balance between genetic, constitutional and cultural factors. The shaping of each person's sexual identity as a complex mixture of those three factors seems to depend to quite a large extent on positive reinforcement or negative aversion stimuli operating in quite subtle ways over the first 20 or so years of life. While the idea of Freud's search for single traumatic events has a superficial attraction about it and while most clinicians can remember a patient where this appears to have been important as a pathogenic agent, it is striking that disturbance as an outcome of rape or incest is by no means inevitable.

The passive absorption of family and social attitudes over many years is likely to be a major influence on final sexual identity. However, there is no doubt that some people have the most extreme sexual feelings and needs which cannot be explained on the basis of their past experience or cultural background and which seem to be an expression of innate personality. It is important to realize just how wide the concept of normality must be spread to include all the common sexual practices elucidated by Kinsey (Kinsey et al. 1948, 1953).

The range of problems that a family doctor can expect to see during his working life will include large numbers of fears and worries related to essentially normal sexual experiences on the one hand and complex mixtures of interpersonal difficulties which may include conflict with the law, violence and death by murder or suicide, on the other.

It is difficult to know which developmental influences of a specific kind during childhood are important. Psychoanalysts have pondered the effects of seductive behaviour towards children of the same or opposite sex by their parents, and proponents and opponents of nudity have written their fair share, too. Most parents relying on 'common sense' produce children who grow up to be sexually functioning adults with minor anxieties about their sexuality which are flavoured by contemporary culture. We do know that masturbation in male and female children of preschool age and from puberty onwards is a normal, pleasurable and harmless activity. We also know that the ability to have a satisfying continuing sexual relationship with a person of the opposite sex probably depends on having had an accepting, trusting relationship with one's parents in a setting where sex was not something to be programmed out by explicit or implicit conditioning of a religious or other nature.

Adolescence

In adolescence, with its confusing mixture of rapid physical growth associated with disturbing changes of body-image, the powerful awakening of sexual feelings and their exploitation by commerce, and the shedding of childhood status for the rewards and responsibilities of adult life are accompanied by fears of inadequacy and potential failure. These fears centre on such things as early or late menarche or growth of pubic hair, breast or penis size, as compared in the showers at school, and the spotty skin and body odour/halitosis so important to the manufacturers of cosmetics and deodorants. For most teenagers, these are minor worries and reassurance is derived from their universality. To a minority, lacking in confidence and a sense of their own value, this can be the beginning of a lonely road to social isolation. It is surprising how many girls develop a transient form of anorexia nervosa with secondary amenorrhoea at this age.

Conflicts over masturbation and homosexual feelings towards teachers or friends usually give way to the conflict over whether or not to have heterosexual intercourse. At this point again, most negotiate the developmental phase, some drift into a lifetime of lonely solitary masturbation, others embark on a pattern of homosexual relationships which they will retain as adults. It is also common to find late teenagers who may have had homosexual and heterosexual relationships and who feel guilty (often about both) asking their family doctor for advice. A denial of the validity of their homosexual experience is probably the commonest response in this situation; it is likely to be the response of least use, since what is needed is somebody to listen in an accepting way and reflect back to the patient the way he appears to be feeling about his dilemma. Any passing of moral judgment is likely to result in further confusion and guilt on the part of the patient, and makes it less likely that he will decide for himself as an adult what is right for him. The danger is that the doctor will accept the parent role and tell the patient as a child what is good for him, thereby perpetuating the patient's child status.

Case History 1

A 29-year-old civil servant was worried that he might be homosexual because the only stimuli which caused him to become erotically aroused were males, both people he knew and film stars he saw when he went to the cinema. He was an only child and his mother died from carcinoma of the breast when he was eight years old. He went to live with three maiden aunts and an unmarried uncle and saw little of his father, who was portrayed as a tough person. When he was 15 years old his father found him masturbating and read him the riot act about his stomach turning to sawdust, etc. At the same time he discovered that his father was having an affair with a woman whose husband was dying. His confusion about sex and his own sexual identity was compounded by the fact that the only other male he knew at that time was a tough army uncle. His feelings then had been that if this was what men were like, he did not feel like a man.

He was referred for psychotherapy over a six-month period, and during this time his self-confidence improved enormously. Whereas before he had always refused invitations to go out with a mixed group from work, he now went out regularly and had played the piano in a pub. He overcame his inability to urinate in a public urinal, was promoted at work (a promotion that had eluded him for several years), and began to be attracted to girls. He himself had terminated his psychotherapy when he felt ready to stand on his own feet.

Adult Dysfunction Causing Patient Distress

Sexual dysfunction in the adult usually presents as an aspect of disturbed interpersonal relationships which may be either causing the problem or be the result of it. In any event the vicious circle of anxiety and recrimination, once set up, aggravates the problem. Commonly, the presentation is that of difficulty in achieving sexual intercourse that is satisfying to both partners in a heterosexual relationship. The complaint may be of loss of interest in sex, impotence or premature ejaculation in the male, vaginismus or failure to climax in the female.

Management

All these problems can be either primary or secondary, and probably the most effective approach to treatment is along the lines developed by Masters and Johnson (1966) as described by Helen Singer Kaplan (1975). This approach is based on behaviourist learning theories and aims to extinguish attitudes and sexual responses which have been developed through years of conditioning, and to replace them with an acceptance of sexuality and a spontaneity in sexual relations.

The treatment involves about 10 half-hour joint consultations (couple plus doctor and another counsellor of the opposite sex), with the couple undertaking to work their way through a series of exercises together between sessions. They are initially barred from attempting intercourse at all, but are told instead to set aside three half-hour periods together during the week when they can explore each other's naked bodies in a comfortable setting. The purpose of this is to defuse the goal-orientated situation which has built up and to create a situation where they can begin to trust each other and to share feelings about their own sexual response. At first only non-genital touching is allowed and the couple is encouraged to discover what is pleasurable to each other. They are encouraged to tell each other what they like and do not like done, so that it becomes possible to say that they do not like something, without the statement being interpreted as a rejection, and to say that they do like something, without it necessarily leading to intercourse. The consultations are used as feedback sessions to examine the feelings that have been generated by the exercises and to look at the resistance to proceed, such as might be demonstrated by a failure to find time for the exercises during the week. Above all else it is vital that the couple should be motivated to achieve a satisfactory adjustment to each other; if this is not the case, then marriage guidance counselling may be more appropriate.

From the dynamic point of view, a number of different things are occurring simultaneously.

1. By coming together for help, the couple are likely to be demonstrating their commitment to each other. When this is not so, it becomes apparent early on and must be brought into the open, as it is futile to embark on treatment with reluctant people. When commitment is present, it creates the basis for the development or the rebuilding of trust.

2. The acceptance of the problem as a legitimate one, deserving of help by a doctor, is itself often the first step towards learning that sex is 'OK', that it is acceptable and can be talked about freely between adults and that it is to be enjoyed. This implies an acceptance by the doctor of the couple's adult sexuality, an acceptance which they themselves may have failed to reach, resulting in their belief that sexual feelings are 'naughty'.

3. The removal of intercourse as an end point, until the couple feel that they both wish to proceed, has a dramatic effect on tensions between the partners. The rediscovery or discovery of non-sexual tenderness is in some ways akin to a return to courtship, laying down the feeling of trust and familiarity with each other's bodies which is the basis for more intimate physical expression.

4. The use of the interviews to discuss feelings, to feedback on how the exercises have progressed without any pressure to go on and please the therapists is an essential first step in the couple taking charge of their own sexual and other feelings and being able to use them creatively with each other.

While primary dysfunction is usually a consequence of a person's background, secondary dysfunctions usually occur in people of brittle adjustment under conditions of some additional stress (e.g. after childbirth or after some years of marriage when the partners have perhaps grown apart and stopped communicating), intercourse having become more of an occasional physiological need rather than an extension of the couple's communications with each other. Inevitably it is rather artificial to consider sexual function in isolation, and it becomes necessary to discuss other aspects of the couple's relationship as they raise them.

When the problem is premature ejaculation, the couple should be instructed in the use of the squeeze technique to delay the male climax. As an exercise the woman should bring the man to the point of climax when he should tell her that he is ready, and she should then squeeze his penis firmly between thumb and first finger just behind the glans; this results in a loss of the urgency to ejaculate and stimulation can begin again. If this is done several times as an exercise, it soon results in a much greater control during intercourse.

With vaginismus, it is usually necessary early in the exercises to encourage the woman to explore her own body and in particular to examine her clitoris and the inside of her vagina by using a mirror. The recommendation to buy one of the well-illustrated books on sexual problems, such as that by David Delvin (1974), is often useful at this stage in bringing about an acceptance that the sexual parts of the body are not 'dirty'. Encouragement to examine the vagina by inserting initially one, later two, and then three fingers is the most natural way for a woman to convince herself that there is room for a penis and that once it is there it will not hurt.

There are many sexual problems of the kind mentioned here that are so severe by the time they present that the most apropriate action is referral to the local psychosexual clinic. However, if the family doctor is receptive in his family planning and postnatal clinics, he will find many of these problems at an early stage, when a relatively small time commitment will achieve a good result and grateful patients. If a doctor decides to develop the use of the Masters and Johnson treatment in his practice, he needs to make the decision as to whether he should treat couples on his own or whether he should involve another member of the primary care team as his co-therapist. In this case, the health visitor or social worker is likely to be the obvious choice, although increasingly marriage guidance counsellors have become involved with this work.

In passing, it is worth remembering that the sexual needs of the disabled and of the elderly are likely to be the same as those of everybody else, although an acceptance of this seems slow. It is also important to inform patients when they are prescribed medication which may affect their sexual feelings or performance. There are still very many people receiving repeat prescriptions for methyldopa which makes them impotent, which they accept as inevitable.

Case History 2

An 18-year-old student returned from France and attended the surgery complaining of diarrhoea. On direct questioning it became apparent that he had had diarrhoea while on holiday, but it had almost settled. When he was challenged he admitted that the real reason for his attendance was impotence of three weeks' duration. His impotence had begun after he had been unfaithful to his girlfriend and now that he had returned from his holiday he would be seeing her again. A ban on intercourse and instruction to restrict himself to petting was agreed upon. When he returned the following week, he reported that he had been so relaxed that he had had a good erection from petting and that they had gone on to intercourse anyway.

Case History 3

A middle-aged couple complained of the husband's premature ejaculation. The couple had been happily married for a long time and their children were grown up. It was the discovery by the mother that her daughter's sex life was more satisfying than her own that had led to her persuading her husband to seek help. Instruction on the squeeze technique and general discussion about their attitudes towards sex was accompanied by the report of a considerable improvement.

Case History 4

A couple in their mid-twenties complained that the wife had lost interest in sex since the birth of their baby two years before. It seemed that the woman had always had mixed feelings about sex but had been able to accept it provided that it was related to childbearing. Her husband had not been as much support to her with the baby as she would have wished, and from a normal initial puerperal loss of interest in sex, the reinforcement of their deteriorating relationship, together with her decision that she wanted no more children if this was what it was like, had aggravated the situation further. However, they were determined that they did want to make the relationship work. A course of 10 interviews with a Masters and Johnson schedule resulted in a resumption of intercourse at a much more satisfying level than previously.

Case History 5

A couple in their early thirties complained of an inability to have intercourse on account of the wife's vaginismus. During an eventful life she had been neglected by her father and had had an illegitimate child during a promiscuous period after leaving home. She loved her husband but wished he would be more assertive and perhaps even cruel to her; if she was in the company of men friends who were more assertive, she would become sexually aroused.

Despite complex psychopathology, a course of some 12 half-hour appointments and a Masters and Johnson regimen resulted in a more assertive husband, much more communication in the relationship and satisfying intercourse for both partners.

Sexual Dysfunction Causing Society Distress

The attitude of society towards sexual behaviour considered deviant today has fluctuated wildly over the centuries and between countries. At present we happen to be in a tolerant period; adulterers are no longer stoned to death, although masturbation is still a crime in some states of the USA. Sexual intercourse before and outside marriage is widespread and accepted and homosexuality is rapidly coming to be accepted as part of the normal range of behaviour.

Exhibitionism

The commonest behaviour which conflicts with the law is exhibitionism (the offence is called indecent exposure). Every year there are about 3,000 convictions in the UK for this offence which occurs in all social classes and at all levels of IQ. There are said to be two types of exhibitionist (Rooth 1971). Type 1 is an inhibited young man of good personality who struggles with his impulse; he exposes a flaccid penis without masturbating and derives little pleasure from the act. The type 2 exhibitionist is more sociopathic. In a state of excitement he exposes an erect penis and masturbates. He derives great pleasure from his behaviour and feels no remorse afterwards. A sadistic element is said to be quite common.

It seems that for many young men, exhibitionism is no more than an expression of sexual frustration and immaturity. Most seem to grow out of it and those who appear in court usually do so only once. The court appearance itself has a marked effect on their behaviour. However, once an exhibitionist has appeared in court twice, he is likely to become a recurrent offender, the compulsive nature of his behaviour being too difficult for him to control.

Most exhibitionists represent no danger to the community, but are rather a nuisance and an embarrassment to their families. Some do go on to more serious offences. This seems to be more likely when the victim is touched during the offence. The problem is that of predicting those who are likely to progress to rape or even murder. An important part of any doctor's management of exhibitionists must be to build up a relationship of trust such that when impulses are building up, the patient is more likely to talk about them in advance.

Patients who have the more worrying pattern of offences may remain as outpatients of the regional forensic psychiatrist but, as these specialists are few, it is common for patients to be returned to their family doctor's care at some stage, often on some form of anti-androgenic preparation, such as cyproterone acetate (Androcur) or an oestrogen. The advantage of the newer cyproterone preparation is that it has fewer side-effects than oestrogens. This is in fact a mixed blessing, because the gynaecomastia produced by oestrogens was the most reliable way of telling whether the patient was taking his medication. The anti-androgens often dramatically affect libido, and the mainstay of treatment is likely to be a combination of one of these with regular appointments to allow the development of a supporting and trusting relationship.

Case History 6

A 21-year-old youth of limited intelligence was a habitual exhibitionist; he had appeared in court on over 80 occasions! He never touched his victims but exposed a flaccid penis and he denied masturbating after the event. The offences occurred whenever he was under stress at work or at home, and had come to be regarded by all concerned as no more than a nuisance. Management consisted of a regular appointment with the family doctor for a chat to allow an opportunity to discuss any tensions which were building up.

Case History 7

An 18-year-old youth, who was regarded by all in his community as a helpful lad, but something of a loner, had been prosecuted several times for indecent exposure. He would exhibit himself to women in the back lane and masturbate. As a result of the offences he had been required by the magistrate to attend a psychiatrist. The psychiatrist reported that it was seemingly impossible to establish a relationship with the patient who would not talk about the offences at all. He had no other mental disorder that could be defined. Some time later he brutally assaulted and murdered a barmaid.

Paedophilia

Paedophilia is probably the sexual offence which arouses most anger in the general public. The paedophiliacs themselves often appear to be immature, and their behaviour can be seen as that of seeking out an immature sex object in keeping with the maturity level of the offender. The behaviour may be either heterosexual or homosexual and rarely leads to violence (there are about four sexual murders of children each year in the UK).

The treatment consists of hormone therapy and psychotherapy. Patients presenting with this problem to a general practitioner should be referred to a psychiatrist for assessment.

Incest

Incest is probably more common than is generally appreciated. It may be tolerated within the family and only come to the attention of outside agencies when a member of the family is referred for another reason. It is probably a symptom of family disturbance and psychiatric referral for a family assessment is indicated.

Rape

Rape is largely a crime committed by young men and second offences are rare. It is perhaps indicative of our cultural values that writers on the subject discuss the rapist but tend to ignore the victim. From the family doctor's point of view, it is the victim who is likely to seek help. Irrespective of whether she played any role in encouraging her assailant, she is likely to be profoundly distressed for some time afterwards. Notwithstanding the physical violence which often accompanies the offence, the victim is likely to feel unclean, especially if prudish, and a sympathetic ear should enable a cathartic expression of feelings to occur. The recent change in the law which allows anonymity of victims in rape cases is likely to encourage more people to come forward for help. It is important that traditional male myths about the role of the victim in rape should not prevent the doctor from providing adequate support.

Fetishism

Fetishism, at one extreme, blends into normal fashion and the display of mating behaviour. At the other extreme, there seems to be a specific learnt association between particular garments and sexual arousal. The discovery of a partner's propensity is likely to precipitate a crisis in the relationship, and it is at such times that the family doctor may be consulted by a confused woman. Generally fetishism is harmless and if other aspects of the relationship are harmonious, the most appropriate action may be to encourage the woman to accept the man for what he is.

Where there is a good clinical psychology service, it may be appropriate to refer for assessment with a view to deconditioning treatment.

Homosexuality

Homosexuality, defined as the experience of being erotically attracted to a member of the same sex, is extremely common. Kinsey (1948) found that more than one third of men admitted to some adult homosexual experience defined as homosexual practice with another man to orgasm. It is likely that his figures were augmented by the inclusion of bisexuals and that the incidence of exclusive homosexual males and females is around four per cent. Genetic studies suggest that there is probably some hereditary component, but how this operates and whether it does so via general personality characteristics is obscure. In any event, it seems likely that patterns of rearing children are more important in the development of sexual propensities.

The increase in society's tolerance of homosexuals over the past few years, and the aggressive attitude of homosexuals who have 'come out' against doctors who label them as deviant, should not deter doctors from noting that homosexuals are at risk for isolation, alcoholism, drug abuse, depression and suicide. Whether these are cause or effect is irrelevant to the awareness of this as a high-risk group in one's practice.

References

Comfort, A., *The Anxiety Makers,* Panther Books, London, 1968.

Delvin, D., *The Book of Love*, New English Library, London, 1974.

Kaplan, H. S., *The Illustrated Manual of Sex Therapy*, Souvenir Press, London, 1975.

Kinsey, A. C., Pomeroy, W. B. and Martine, C. E., *Sexual Behaviour in the Human Male*, W. B. Saunders, Philadelphia and London, 1948.

Kinsey, A. C., Pomeroy, W. B., Martine, C. E. and Gebhard, P. H., *Sexual Behaviour in the Human Female,* W. B. Saunders, Philadelphia and London, 1953.

Masters, W. H. and Johnson, V. E., *Human Sexual Response*, Little Brown, Boston, 1966.

Rooth, F. G., *Br. J. Hosp. Med.*, 1971, **5**, 521.

Further Reading

Brecher, E. M., *The Sex Researchers*, André Deutsch, London, 1970.

Gunn, J., *Br. J. Hosp. Med.*, 1976, **15**, 57.

Schofield, M., *The Sexual Behaviour of Young People*, Pelican, Harmondsworth, 1968.

Storr, A., *Sexual Deviation*, Pelican, Harmondsworth, 1974.

West, D. J., *Homosexuality,* Pelican, Harmondsworth, 1968.

9. Aspects of Fertility and Abortion

Until very recently the roles of women as childbearers and of men as wage-earners were unchallenged. Consequently, a woman's adult identity was related to her feelings about birth and childrearing to an extent which is already beginning to seem extreme. However, strongly held views about the role of women still dominate discussion, and the emotional investment in particular patterns of behaviour and feelings is such that most people know what is best for everybody else even when they are not very sure what is best for themselves.

Psychological disturbances of reproductive life are surrounded by their own mythologies and folk explanations which are still widely subscribed to today. However, the recent infatuation of doctors with the scientific method as it relates to 'hard' science has led to attempts to explain away disturbances in terms of theories based on biochemistry and physiology. What is really needed is some unifying theory which takes account of the subtleties of human emotion and the intimate relationship of the mood centres of the hypothalamus to the adjacent centres which regulate the secretion of sex hormones.

Whilst epidemiological perspectives may throw light on themes and modes of function by referring to populations of patients, ultimately the meaning of fertility to an individual and its psychosomatic aspects can only be made sense of in the light of the patient's own story.

Menstruation and Premenstrual Tension

If, to some women, menstruation is an unpleasant ritual inflicted upon them every month, to others it is an accepted manifestation of their sex and potential fertility. For many others a period is received with relief as a sign of pregnancy avoided. The premenstrual tension syndrome occurs in as many as 10 per cent of all women. Irritability and depression with weeping for no apparent reason may be marked, and there may be nausea, migrainous headache, dizziness and disturbance of appetite, sleep and sexual desire. For some women the pelvic discomfort and pain of dysmenorrhoea may be the main focus of complaint.

Premenstrual women are over-represented in sickness absence, acute admissions to psychiatric hospital and crimes of violence committed by women, as well as accidents, suicide and attempted suicide.

Explanations have concentrated on the interactions of hormone changes with electrolyte disturbance or the premorbid personality of sufferers. It has proved very difficult to define the nature of supposed biological changes and clarification awaits further work. The general practice study by Kessel and Coppen (1963) found a significant correlation between premenstrual symptoms and neuroticism.

Simple analgesics and sedatives are probably the most usually prescribed remedies, whilst diuretics and combined preparations of oestrogen and progestogen are sometimes of value if given during the last few days of the cycle.

Unfortunately, menstruation can quite easily become the focus for vague and ill-defined uneasiness about sex-role and identity and, whilst many such fears are of a transient developmental nature, some women develop a self-reinforcing fear of menstruation which affects the lives of themselves and those around them and which in turn influences their daughters' attitude to their bodies and to sex. Simple explanation, sympathetic listening and reassurance at an early stage may have the desired effect, but in established sufferers it may well serve as a reward for a symptom which has become part of a strategy of life.

Contraception

The apparently willing participation of doctors as generators of anxiety and guilt has been well documented by Alex Comfort (Comfort 1968). Contraception has been one area where doctors have never appeared to be lost for an opinion, and in the early part of the century it was commonly held to be an unnatural practice which could lead to a variety of medical conditions. The last 20 years have seen the widespread acceptance of contraceptive practice by all social groups and by members of most religions, even when their leaders continue to oppose it.

Between 1970 and 1975 the proportion of married women relying on oral contraception increased from 20 to 36 per cent. It is this group of women who are of most interest from the point of view of psychological reactions since, with one exception, there is no intrinsic cause for psychological disturbance from any of the other commonly used forms of contraception. The exception is withdrawal which, apart from being unreliable as a method of contraception, requires a degree of self-control which is unlikely to be acquired without considerable experience and the risk of unwanted pregnancy. It is probable that this method, which is still quite widely practised, leads to frustration, particularly on the part of women, and to consequent marital dissatisfaction and a failure to optimize the value of sexual intercourse within a relationship.

Mild symptoms of depression, irritability and loss of libido appear to be quite common amongst women taking oral contraceptives. The evidence for a causal relationship is far from clear and studies have had conflicting findings. Whilst for some women psychiatric symptoms seem to occur, for others oral contraception seems to lead to a sense of wellbeing, increased libido and an alleviation of premenstrual tension and depression. There is some suggestion that the more strongly oestrogenic pills are most likely to cause mental disturbance.

Opinion varies as to the possible aetiology of psychiatric disturbance. There are those who believe that it represents an inner conflict of the woman in preventing pregnancy, whilst others have suggested that oral contraceptives interfere with tryptophan and monoamine oxidase metabolism and therefore with mood regulation by way of the hypothalamic centres. Faced with such conflicting facts, explanations which take account of constitutional and psychological factors in individual women are likely to be of most heuristic value in the consulting room.

Pregnancy and Childbirth

Anxiety in pregnancy is a normal phenomenon. All would-be parents worry that their child may be abnormal or that things may go wrong, and concern over the change of life style which will follow a first pregnancy is a realistic one. If the pregnancy is unwanted or the mother's attitude towards it is one of ambivalence, then greater problems of adjustment are to be anticipated. Ambivalence to pregnancy has been especially implicated in the aggravation of hyperemesis.

For many women, producing children is still the only creative outlet open to them. Their success in carrying out this task, and how others, perhaps in particular their mothers, judge their ability are taken very seriously. Worries and fears such as these could be discussed at the antenatal clinic given an opening and a relaxed atmosphere; the health visitor or practice nurse has important prophylactic potential here.

The change in the social climate which has reduced the pressure on women to have children whether they want them or not, together with the increased information, preparation for childbirth and tolerance of consorts in the delivery suite are all developments which might be expected to have reduced the stress of pregnancy. However, the increasing medicalization of pregnancy in terms of levels of hospital confinement and the increasing isolation of the nuclear family are probably acting in the opposite direction.

Some men experience an unusual degree of identification with their wives during pregnancy to the extent of acquiring symptoms of pregnancy themselves. This may not be uncommon to a mild extent but when it is severe—the so-called couvade syndrome—the level of tension involved may require treatment with anxiolytic drugs. The prognosis is benign, although the condition tends to occur in future pregnancies.

Despite the changes of metabolism and endocrine function in pregnancy, there is no increased risk of major mental illness and for many neurotic women, pregnancy is a remarkably healthy and trouble-free time. Patients who have experienced an affective disorder in the past may have a relapse during pregnancy, and this can be treated effectively with ECT without ill-effect to the child. Established schizophrenia is usually unaffected by pregnancy but when it is, with careful management the pregnancy can be brought to term uneventfully. The option of termination of the pregnancy should be considered in the context of the woman's total situation and her ability to look after a child fully with the usual community support.

Suicidal attempts in pregnancy are not uncommon, especially when the pregnancy is unwanted. Suicide does occur in pregnancy despite claims to the contrary.

Major psychiatric illness follows about one birth in 1,000 and there is an increased psychiatric admission rate for affective disorder in the first few months following birth. When a breakdown occurs, the clinical picture is frequently mixed and may include some clouding of consciousness. Insomnia, depression or elation, disturbed thoughts, perception and ideas are not uncommon. The distinction between affective disorder and schizophrenia may be difficult and the definitive diagnosis may need to be postponed. The distinction between a primary functional disorder and an organic one, such as may arise from a thromboembolus or puerperal sepsis, may be important.

The most common time for developing psychiatric disturbance after childbirth is within two weeks of the birth. It is probable that most illnesses developing within three months postpartum are precipitated by childbirth, whilst those arising during pregnancy or later in the postpartum period are largely coincidental.

Treatment of a major disorder will require hospitalization and fortunately most Health Authorities now have provision for admitting the mother and baby together. ECT followed by antidepressant medication may be required for an acute affective disorder and depot phenothiazines for one to two years for a schizophrenic breakdown.

Apart from the major disorders occurring after childbirth, it is common for women to develop mild depression or postpartum 'blues'. Whilst major disorders appear to be constitutionally allied to major disorders occurring at other times, the pregnancy acting as a trigger mechanism, less severe levels of disturbance are more likely to be related to psychological adjustment to the birth or to hormone changes. Obsessional and overdependent women are said to be more prone to disturbance at this time.

Although it is possible that the prognosis for affective disorder is worse when it occurs postpartum than when it occurs at other times, the improvement in prognosis in recent years with modern therapies contrasts markedly with that previously when many of these patients spent the remainder of their lives in the back-wards of mental hospitals. The prognosis of postpartum schizophrenia is variable and, as with schizophrenia arising at other times, it must be a guarded one.

Abortion

The 1967 Abortion Act was a landmark in British social legislation. Some saw it as the hallmark of a civilized society, whilst for others it marked the decline of morality, which they believed to be occurring all around them. However, Sir George Godber and other prominent medical figures, such as Sir Dougal Baird, have had little doubt of its potential impact on the welfare of women (Godber 1969; Baird 1975). The evidence to support this view comes from studies which demonstrate a strong link between unwanted and illegitimate pregnancy and raised perinatal mortality rates on the one hand, and a range of social pathologies, including alcoholism, delinquency and psychiatric disorder in unwanted children, on the other.

Before the Act it was estimated that between 100,000 and 200,000 illegal abortions were performed annually (Ferris 1966). Subsequently, the number of legal abortions has levelled off at 100,000 to 110,000 per annum, and there is little doubt that illegal abortion in the UK is now uncommon (Tietze and Murstein 1975).

It is common to suppose that abortion must have a profound effect on the mother. However, Jeffcoate's view that 'a significant proportion of women, sometimes rated at 20 to 30 per cent in the past, are adversely affected emotionally throughout their life' is not supported by well planned studies (Jeffcoate 1970). Systematic follow-up has found remarkably few serious psychiatric sequelae following abortion and when they do occur, they are usually related to longstanding emotional difficulties.

When psychological reactions occur they usually relate to feelings of guilt or regret and are short-lived. The factors determining a satisfactory outcome seem to be those which are conducive to a woman making a decision which she believes to be her own in a context where she is accorded respect and support. The presence of ambivalence, coercion, a medical indication or concomitant severe psychiatric illness carry a poorer prognosis, whilst the attitudes of lay and professional contacts during the operation period may influence the outcome.

Adequate counselling of women requesting abortion includes a discussion of the alternatives open to them with no attempt by the doctor to force his own moral or ethical views on his patient. If he feels unable to participate in abortion counselling from a neutral position, he should explain this to his patient so that she can seek alternative counselling and gynaecological referral if this is required.

Sadly, it seems that women cannot currently rely on neutral counselling, support or even necessarily respect from the doctors they consult when they wish to have an abortion (Ashton 1978).

Delays which occur as the result of family doctors not making their ethical objection to abortion and their unwillingness to refer to a gynaecologist explicit to their patients can make the difference between patients having relatively simple first trimester operations or more hazardous second trimester operations. The ambivalence and uncertainty which is caused in women caught in their doctors' dilemmas can then cause guilt feelings which would have been unlikely if they had been handled more sympathetically.

Studies of mothers and their children when request for abortion has been turned down show a high incidence of regrets and resentment by the mothers and of psychiatric disturbance, delinquency, educational under-achievement and poor work records for the offspring (Forssman and Thuwe 1966).

Sterilization

The growth in the demand for both male and female sterilization has taken most people by surprise. Increasingly, childbearing is felt to be something which should occur before the age of 30 years, and couples faced with the prospect of 20 years' contraception are preferring to opt for one or other partner to be sterilized. Fears that such a permanent step will be regretted later do not appear to be supported when the decision has been made after careful thought.

Female Sterilization

When a woman genuinely wishes to be sterilized and fully understands and has considered the consequences, the outcome from the point of view of psychological adjustment is remarkably good. However, when there is any question of coercion or if the operation is being carried out for medical indications and the woman would really have liked to have had further pregnancies, quite serious regrets may occur.

·All women requesting sterilization require careful counselling and this is particularly true of younger women. In one study, women under 26 years of age who are sterilized were much less likely to be satisfied with the operation (Ekblad 1961).

For many women the removal of the fear of pregnancy and anxieties about the use of oral contraception seem to lead to improved sexual responsiveness and satisfaction.

Male Sterilization

Men seem to be much more likely to regard their virility and potency as being one and the same thing than do women, and for this reason many men will not contemplate vasectomy.

However, when a man agrees to the operation of his own free will and without duress, the outcome is usually extremely good. Frequently, potency and satisfaction with intercourse are reported to have improved after the operation and in one series only 18 out of 1,011 operations led to dissatisfaction with the operation by one or both partners (Jackson 1969).

Menopause

The commonly occurring symptoms of the menopause include irritability, depression and weepiness, insomnia, fainting and dizziness. The actual mechanism for these symptoms remains conjectural, and it is probable that adjustment to the developmental crisis which the menopause marks is at least as important as the endocrine changes.

Treatment with oestrogens, sedatives and general support are the most practicable forms of help and it is important not to overlook the physical conditions which may develop in middle life and be ignored as menopausal symptoms.

Affective disorders, which seem particularly likely to occur at this time, require full assessment, and if necessary, treatment with adequate dosage of antidepressant medication or admission for inpatient treatment.

References

Ashton, J. R., Induced Abortion in the Wessex Health Region: The Provision and Utilization of Services, M.SC Thesis, London School of Hygiene, 1978.

Baird, D., *J. Med. Ethic.*, 1975, **1**, 122.

Comfort, A., *The Anxiety Makers*, Panther Books, London, 1968.

Ekblad, M., *Acta Psychiat. Scand.*, 1961, Suppl. 161.

Ferris, P., *The Nameless—Abortion in Britain Today*, Hutchinson, London, 1966.

Forssman, H. and Thuwe, I., *Acta Psychiat. Scand.*, 1966, **42**, 71.

Godber, G. E., *Lancet*, 1969, **ii**, 312.

Jackson, L. N., *Practitioner*, 1969, **203**, 320.

Jeffcoate, T. N. A., *'Abortion' in Morals and Medicine*, BBC Publications, London, 1970.

Kessel, W. I. N. and Coppen, A., *Lancet*, 1963, **ii**, 61.

Tietze, C. and Murstein, M. C., *Induced Abortion*, 1975 Factbook, Population Council, London, 1975.

Further Reading

Enoch, B., Trethowan, W. H. and Barker, J.C., *Some Uncommon Psychiatric Syndromes*, John Wright, Bristol, 1967.

Pitt, B., Psychiatric illness following childbirth, in *Contemporary Psychiatry: Selected Reviews from the British Journal of Hospital Medicine*, Trevor Silverstone and Brian Barraclough (Eds), Headley Bros, Ashford, 1975.

Tonks, C. M., Premenstrual tension, in *Contemporary Psychiatry: Selected Reviews from the British Journal of Hospital Medicine*, Trevor Silverstone and Brian Barraclough (Eds), Headley Bros, Ashford, 1975.

10. Alcohol and Drug Abuse

'Through ages man's desires,
to free his mind to release his very soul
have proved to all who live,
that death itself is freedom for ever more,
and your troubled young life will make you turn,
to the needle of death'

(Bert Jansch)

Introduction

There is little doubt that the use of psychoactive drugs for non-medicinal purposes has long been a universal phenomenon and the ingenuity which man has applied to producing pharmacologically active substances commands respect. These have ranged from the fermentation products of barley, moss and coconut milk, to extracts of mushrooms, cactus and poppies. To a large extent, the local substance is enshrined in the culture and takes its place in the ecology of social life with taboos and sanctions alongside formalized use in religious or everyday rites.

In recent years the rapid changes in mobility have led to a cross-fertilization of cultural ideas, which has resulted in our exporting whisky and beer in association with religious guilt, and importing marijuana and a variety of exotic equivalents with reggae music, meditation and carry-out curries. To some extent this is such a recent phenomenon that it has the characteristics of a generation effect and the over-35s have very little idea how to respond to habits which succeeding generations have either integrated into their life style or towards which they have at least defined their own attitudes from the basis of their own or others' observed experience. Consequently, the subject of drugs tends to generate a great deal of heat and emotion and very little light or rational thought.

On the one hand, we seem to view with equanimity an epidemic of alcoholism and dependence on prescribed tranquillizers and, on the other, we seem happy to ignore the alienation of large sectors of the younger population who have been prosecuted and stigmatized with all the authority of the law for using cannabis, about which we have surprisingly little scientific data, mainly because we are unwilling to face up to the issues involved if it should prove to be at least as 'harmless' as alcohol, as many people have suggested. The ensuing confusion over drugs and the subsequent ineffectiveness of the law to control narcotics, which extract a small but definite annual toll of our youth, are matters for some concern.

The Nature of Dependence

The use of the term 'addiction' in drug abuse was dropped by the World Health Organization in 1964 because of the difficulty of distinguishing it from what was known as drug habituation (habit). Instead, the concept of 'dependence' was introduced, being 'a state, sometimes psychic and sometimes also physical, resulting from the interaction between a living organism and a drug, characterized by behavioural and other responses that always include a compulsion to take the drug on a continuous or periodic basis in order to experience its psychic effects and sometimes to avoid the discomfort of its absence. Tolerance may not be present. A person may be dependent on more than one drug.'

Psychic Dependence

In all types of drug dependence there is psychic dependence characterized by a psychological need to continue to take the drug, but with some drugs, particularly morphine, barbiturates and alcohol, there are actually physiological consequences of stopping the drug which are reversed when it is once again taken in adequate dose. The extent of the overlap between psychic and physical dependence can be difficult to confirm in the individual case, although the transition from one state to the other may be quite dramatic.

Tolerance

Dependence is also characterized by the propensity for tolerance to develop, which is indicated by a reduced effect from a given dose of the drug and a progressive increase in the quantity taken. Lawrence (1966) reminds us that 'it is probable that any drug that alters consciousness can be a subject of dependence', and it is worth bearing this in mind when new preparations are introduced as being non-dependence producing.

Types of Drug Dependence

The WHO Expert Committee on Drug Dependence defined eight groups of dependence-producing drugs:

1. Morphine type.
2. Barbiturate type.
3. Alcohol type (affinity with barbiturate type).

4. Amphetamine type.

5. Cocaine type.

6. Cannabis type.

7. Hallucinogenic type.

8. Khat type.

Khat is a leaf found in South Yemen and the Horn of Africa and it is chewed to obtain the desired effect. It is not usually encountered in this country and will not be discussed further here.

Morphine-type Dependence

The term morphine-type dependence covers the group of drugs based on opium and its derivatives, morphine and heroin, and the many semisynthetic and synthetic substances with morphine-like effects, including methadone, pethidine and dextromoramide. This group of drugs commonly has properties of physical, as well as psychic, dependence and when they are withdrawn suddenly, a variety of disturbances, mainly mediated through the autonomic nervous system, occur. These effects are especially common after heroin withdrawal and range from yawning, perspiration, lacrimation and rhinorrhoea to disturbances of respiration, blood pressure and gastrointestinal function; they are accompanied by persistent restlessness and craving for the drug (Table 14).

Table 14. Symptoms of withdrawal in morphine-type dependence.

Yawning

Perspiration

Lacrimation

Rhinorrhoea

Restlessness

Mydriasis

Anorexia

Insomnia

Hypertension

Pyrexia

Tachycardia

Vomiting

Diarrhoea

Spontaneous ejaculation

Pattern of Dependence

The past decade has seen a great change in the pattern of dependence in this group. Prior to 1965 there were probably only about 500 people involved throughout the UK; these were usually older people and quite likely to be members of the medical or nursing professions who had begun taking drugs in association with physical illness. Since then, this group of drugs has been used increasingly by younger people with the spread of an international consumer youth culture and the number of users has grown steadily. By 1968 the number of dependent persons known to the Home Office had increased to about 2,500 and it has continued to increase at a steady rate since, although there are disputes as to the actual extent of the numbers currently involved.

Morphine-type addiction seems to have many of the characteristics of a contagious disease and some of the epidemiological studies have defined clear transmission trees tracing back secondary and tertiary cases to a primary source who has introduced friends or associates to the habit. De Alarcon and Rathod carried out an extensive community survey of heroin abuse in Harlow New Town with case identification from local probation and police reports, responses from known heroin users and surveys of recently jaundiced inpatients and casualty admissions for overdoses of hypnotics or stimulants (De Alarcon and Rathod 1968). They concluded that the prevalence rate was 8.5 per 1,000 of those aged 15 to 25 years.

A complicating factor has been the existence of a few doctors who, for one reason or another, have been sympathetic to 'junkies' and have prescribed excessive quantities of narcotics before the freedom to do so was restricted.

The propensity to morphine-type dependency is not, as is commonly supposed, related to social class, although it has been suggested that there is a significant tendency for the subjects to have parents in the professions. The families of those dependent on heroin show an excess of psychiatric disturbance and other dependencies including alcohol and criminal behaviour.

The subjects themselves have often demonstrated antisocial and unstable personalities with poor school and work records antedating their dependence. Once the dependence is established, criminal association is much more likely in view of the high cost of sustaining the habit unless they become registered with a Home Office recognized doctor. Male and female prostitution is common as a method of raising money.

The establishment of dependence and the ensuing association with a tight group of like-minded people is rapidly consolidated by the bewilderment, hostility and outright rejection by families and straight society. Thus the downward spiral path towards poor living conditions and nutrition and withdrawal from meaningful interpersonal relationships becomes established. The maintenance of the habit assumes priority over all other needs, and varying degrees of malnutrition impair the normal capacity to cope with the repeated intercurrent infections which are a consequence of the life style. In addition septic injection sites and abscesses, syringe transmitted jaundice and syphilis and accidental or deliberate overdose are regular hazards. The mortality rate is of the order of 30 per 1,000 per annum in the UK compared with 1 per 1,000 for the general population of the same age.

Concern over the large increase of morphine-type dependence resulted in the Dangerous Drugs Act 1967 and the Dangerous (Notification of Addicts) Drugs Regulations 1968, which require any doctor to notify the Chief Medical Officer of the Home Office of details of a patient whom he suspects has become 'so dependent upon the drug that he has an overwhelming desire for the administration of it to be continued'. This legislation was accompanied by the Dangerous Drugs (Supply to Addicts) Regulations 1968, which prohibits a medical practitioner from administering or authorizing the administration of cocaine or heroin to drug dependent persons except under licence or for the purpose of relieving pain due to organic disease or injury.

Treatment and Management

Treatment and general management lie with the local psychiatrist with responsibility for drug abuse, and consideration of treatment methods in any detail will not be gone into here. The social prognosis is generally poor since the lack of the very requirements of a good outcome in psychotherapy, namely a good premorbid personality and motivation, are amongst the factors which predispose to drug dependence in the first place. The general practitioner needs to be aware of the syndromes and sequelae of addiction in this group so that he can take such action as may be necessary to minimize the effects.

Barbiturate-type Dependence

It is now generally accepted that there are few indications for barbiturate use in general practice. However, vast numbers of people have been taking them regularly as night sedation or as a tranquillizer for many years, and it would seem that the rational approach is to avoid new prescriptions, to substitute with benzodiazepines where feasible, and to accept that there is a group of older patients who will be taking barbiturates for the rest of their lives.

Barbiturate dependence is similar in character to that of alcohol and withdrawal may be accompanied by a psychosis with fits and even death. This group of drugs has been commonly used by successful suicides. As with most drug abuse in the 1970s, they are not uncommonly injected intravenously by younger people.

Alcohol-type Dependence

The problems of all other forms of drug addiction in the UK pale into insignificance when compared with alcohol. The consequences of pathological drinking affect everybody; the alcoholic, the spouse and children, work colleagues and the rest of society. It is said that the alcoholic is liable to lose his wife, his job and his stomach, and although this is often the case, the impact of alcoholics even without this degree of disturbance is a major social and public health problem.

The Finnish Foundation for Alcohol Studies has concluded that amongst other things, heavy users of alcohol have a substantially elevated risk of premature death and that the aetiological importance of alcohol is clear with respect to death from cirrhosis of the liver, accidents and cancers of the upper respiratory and upper digestive tracts (Finnish Foundation for Alcohol Studies 1975). In addition alcohol abuse has a strong association with crime, violence and suicide, and is a potent aetiological factor in disturbed development in the alcoholic's children.

Unravelling our attitudes towards our own cultural 'poison' is very difficult because we are so close to it; certainly it seems that we bend over backwards to avoid seeing it as a problem and our cultural tolerance of excessive drinking makes consensus over definitions particularly difficult. The *Medical Memorandum on Drug Dependence*, published by the Department of Health, excluded any discussion of alcohol dependence, whilst dealing with all seven other types (DHSS 1972). The WHO defines alcoholics as 'those excessive drinkers whose dependence on alcohol has attained such a degree that they show a noticeable disturbance or an interference with their mental and bodily health, their interpersonal relations and their smooth social and economic functioning, or who show prodromal signs of such development'.

Such a definition at least seeks to put alcohol abuse into operational terms; unfortunately, the conspiracy of silence which so often surrounds alcohol abuse, the cover-up by workmates, the tolerance of excessive consumption of alcohol, which is a characteristic of the medical profession itself, make such factors hard to define.

Jellinek developed and later abandoned a formula for estimating the numbers of alcoholics based on the numbers of deaths per annum from cirrhosis of the liver where alcohol was a factor (Jellinek 1960). However, Jellinek's formula does allow us to conclude that there are at least 350,000 alcoholics in Britain.

Effects of Alcohol

Alcohol affects the nervous system in diverse ways. Apart from the immediate effects of acute intoxication leading to drunkenness, disinhibition, violence, hypoglycaemia and coma, there are the secondary effects of chronic alcoholism on the CNS. The direct effects of chronic alcoholism are to produce lesions of the gastrointestinal tract, including the liver, and the indirect effects include those that occur as a consequence of poor nutrition (malnutrition itself, B group vitamin deficiencies, intercurrent infections and, less commonly now, tuberculosis) and the obscure neurological degenerative diseases, including alcoholic dementia.

Pattern of Dependence

Alcoholism has in the past been more common in men than in women, but this is changing. It probably shows no class preference except inasmuch as the middle classes tend to be able to conceal it for longer, and it is commoner in jobs associated with travel or ready access to free or cheap alcohol. In general terms, the freer the availability of alcohol, the more alcoholics there will be and the less likely they are to be of severely disturbed personality. Single and divorced people, and especially widowers, have high rates of alcoholism, as do children from large families and those later in the birth order. In recent years, in common with all forms of drug abuse, there has been a tendency for younger people to be affected; this is probably in part related to increased purchasing power.

Commonly alcoholics progress in a stepwise fashion from initial intermittent heavy drinking to the persistent, all-day use of nearly neat alcohol, with secret bottles, sessions at lunchtime and night and a bottle to take home to bed. The steps may follow a personal crisis or a period working away from home and it is frequently only when social catastrophe occurs or the courts intervene, that help is sought.

Most family doctors are only aware of a very few of the 25 or 30 alcoholics on their list; even if they were aware of them all, it is likely that many would refuse help and that the resources available would be inadequate to cope with those who were willing to try to deal with their problem. Probably the most realistic course is for the doctor to maintain a watchful eye on those patients whom he suspects of alcohol abuse and to be ready to offer help when a crisis occurs.

It is especially important to consider alcoholism as a cause of acute delirium during abstinence enforced perhaps by an intercurrent infection. This severe, physical withdrawal syndrome, characterized by severe confusion, disordered perception, insomnia, agitation, delusions and hallucinations, is associated with a mortality rate of about 10 per cent.

In patients who are drinking heavily, but who will not stop drinking, it is prudent to keep regular checks on their haematological state with a view to prescribing courses of parenteral vitamins (such as Parentrovite).

Breaking the Habit

Patients sometimes seek help in reducing their drinking whilst not really being prepared to accept that they are dependent. In this situation, it is best to arrive at a joint plan with targets and to provide support by substituting a regular benzodiazepine for some of the alcohol with a view to tailing this off when the drinking is stabilized. Diazepam 5 to 10 mg t.d.s. is an appropriate preparation usually. Heminevrin has advantages in that it is metabolized along the same pathways as alcohol, but it is liable itself to be the subject of dependence, and should probably not be prescribed outside a hospital setting.

When patients reach a crisis point with their drinking, they frequently lack the motivation to deal with the underlying problems in a radical way. For these people, admission to an acute psychiatric unit for 'drying out' is indicated, and this usually requires two to three weeks. Subsequent contact with Alcoholics Anonymous will improve the prognosis.

A small proportion of well-motivated patients benefit from intensive psychotherapy over some months in a specialized unit. Such units are very selective about who they take and even so have a high drop-out rate. In some units the goal of controlled drinking is now aspired to for some patients, as opposed to the AA philosophy of total abstinence.

Prognosis

Overall the prognosis for alcoholics is rather dismal, but in view of the consequences of no intervention, humanitarian considerations require that health workers seek to maintain their optimism.

Amphetamine-type Dependence

There is no justification for prescribing amphetamine group drugs in general practice and these drugs should cease to be a problem in the foreseeable future. In the past, they have been widely used as an aid to slimming and for keeping awake, for example for examination revision or all-night parties. They can lead to the rapid development of psychological dependence, and some people are especially prone to develop a paranoid psychosis when taking them.

Unfortunately, for as long as any patients are prescribed amphetamines, pharmacists will need to stock them and will therefore be a target for break-ins and a source of illicit drug use.

Cocaine-type Dependence

Cocaine abuse is unusual in the UK, although sniffing it seems to have a current vogue amongst pop stars. It produces psychic dependence without physical dependence and without the development of tolerance. Clinically it produces excitation, dilated pupils (contrasting with the pinpoint pupils of heroin), tremors and hallucinations.

Cannabis-type Dependence

There is little doubt that cannabis is now very widely used in the UK and in western countries generally. There is said to be emotional dependence without physical dependence and with the development of only minor tolerance.

The term cannabis itself is usually used to include all the products of the plant *Cannabis sativa*; a plant which is remarkably adaptive and undoubtedly to be found growing unsuspected in the gardens of suburban England in the 1970s. The resinous exudate of the flowering tops tends to be called 'hashish' and the leaves and stalks 'marijuana' or 'grass'. The active ingredient of both is probably a tetrahydrocannabinol.

Use of Cannabis

Cannabis is usually smoked in a social setting by groups of sympathetic people, who pass a 'joint' around, inhaling the smoke into their lungs and holding it there whilst the active component is absorbed. The efficacy of the preparation in producing psychotomimetic effects depends upon the user's previous experience, expectations and personality, and in this respect it is similar to alcohol. Physiologically it produces dilation of the conjunctival vessels, an irritation of the throat, slight increases in the pulse and blood pressure and either great hunger or else a complete lack of interest in food. Psychologically it produces distortions of perception which are generally found to be pleasant, with a more vivid appreciation of sound and colour and a feeling of wellbeing.

It is widely claimed that cannabis facilitates communication and reduces aggressiveness, although opponents of the drug claim that the name 'hashish', being related to 'assassin', is proof of its harmful effects. It is to be hoped that current work will throw some light on this controversy.

When people use cannabis regularly on their own they are very likely to be disturbed in the same way as are solitary alcoholics, but otherwise the suggestion that cannabis smokers are especially abnormal is unsubstantiated, although people who are socially deviant are more likely to smoke cannabis in the same way that they are more likely to smoke anything, to drink alcohol to excess and to be involved in accidents of various sorts.

The problem with cannabis is that our blinkered response to it has led to a punitive and often destructive treatment of users. Our unwillingness to invest in research has led us into a situation where young people who have been told that cannabis is harmful are unlikely to believe that other drugs are harmful, having evaluated cannabis for themselves. Because cannabis is illegal, users are likely to come into contact with other drugs when they come to buy supplies, and in effect the very society that claims to protect them is placing them at risk. What is really needed is objective research and a rational policy based on the facts.

Hallucinogenic-type Dependence

Several synthetic hallucinogenic drugs including LSD (lysergic acid diethylamide) have now achieved widespread use, especially among student communities. These drugs cause a short-lived, psychotic-like state with hallucinations and delusions during which suicide or self-harm may occur. Some people who are predisposed may develop an ongoing psychosis and an unusual feature of this group is the occurrence of 'flashbacks' (recurrences of the 'trip') at a later date, which may be accompanied by great anxiety.

Usually these drugs are taken in a controlled situation in the sense that one person refrains from 'tripping' and looks after the others in case anybody has a 'bad trip'. The management of a bad trip in everyday drug culture involves looking after the person and comforting them; clinically it tends to mean observation in a casualty ward. An LSD trip usually lasts from 6 to 10 hours.

Earlier reports of LSD causing chromosome damage have not been substantiated.

Conclusion

Drug abuse brings to the fore all the problems of defining illness and illness behaviour, not to mention the conflicting perspectives of different generations. Whilst the question of whether drug dependence is an illness has no clear answers, the impact of drug dependence in producing ill health is, in most cases, quite clear.

Our attitudes to drugs are coloured by our own experience and by our cultural background. In an increasingly pluralistic, multiracial community with rapid communication it is unrealistic to reject out of hand the habits of other countries. If our approach to drug abuse is to be rational, we need to examine the evidence in the same way that we would examine it for any other drug before passing judgement.

At the end of the day, drug abuse strategies must be about prevention, education and control, rather than about treatment, for by the time treatment is needed, it is usually too expensive and is unlikely to be effective. Rational strategies of prevention require a clear mind and a willingness to compromise; if cannabis turns out to be less harmful than alcohol, we must see if we are flexible enough to make the necessary adjustments.

References

Bert Jansch, *Needle of Death*, Transatlantic Records.

De Alarcon, R. and Rathod, N. H., *Br. Med. J.*, 1968, **2**, 549.

DHSS, *Medical Memorandum on Drug Dependence*, HMSO, London, 1972.

Finnish Foundation for Alcohol Studies, *Alcohol Control Policies in Public Health Perspective*, Vol. 25, 1972.

Jellinek, E. M., *The Disease Concept of Alcoholism*, Hill House, New Haven, 1960.

Kessel, N. and Walton, H., *Alcoholism*, Penguin, Harmondsworth, 1965.,

Lawrence, D. R., *Clinical Pharmacology*, Churchill, Edinburgh, 1966.

11. Forensic Psychiatry

Human behaviour is infinitely variable and by no means always in the best interests of other members of the community. Consequently, all societies evolve rules which define the limits of acceptable behaviour. Such limits usually relate to offences against property and against the person but there is a third group of offences, such as prostitution and drug abuse, which fall into neither of these categories, but which involve behaviour that society considers delinquent and against the best interests of the community.

The Limits of Acceptable Behaviour

The limits of acceptable behaviour are very much a function of the times and the past two decades have seen the evolution of a much more tolerant and liberal society with a greater emphasis on the freedom of the individual to do as he wishes, as long as his actions do not impinge upon the rights of others. In this respect the liberalization of the laws relating to suicide, homosexuality, abortion and divorce have probably been the most important measures. Simultaneously, we have seen some redefinition of crime, so that people are more likely to be defined as 'ill' rather than 'wicked', and there is great concern that those who transgress the law should not be subject to management which may be more destructive and brutalizing than the crime they have committed. An interest has developed in tightening up the laws governing behaviour which is a threat to others, such as drinking and driving, although in a perverse way it is still half-regarded as a civil right to drive a motor car when incapable of doing so safely.

The Doctor's Responsibility

The general practitioner is likely to be called on for his professional knowledge when one of his patients has come into conflict with the law and there is some question that his mental or physical state has a bearing on the offence. The doctor's concern in these cases is with both the practical clinical care of his patient and with fulfilling his obligation to the community as a responsible citizen. Although general practitioners are not usually psychiatrically trained and therefore not able to provide a detailed clinical report of the patient's mental state, their position as primary physicians and generalists means that they are probably best placed to bring together and interpret the findings from various clinical sources, as well as the social data which provide the essential backcloth to any assessment. When such an assessment is required, it is usually by the Magistrates' court and with the consent of the patient. However, this situation always carries the potential for a conflict of interests.

A doctor's first responsibility is to his patient but, on occasions, he has a wider obligation to the community which overrides this, and in any particular situation it may be extremely difficult to decide on the ethically correct course of action. The practical rule must always be to protect the patient's interests, and information gained in the consulting room should not be divulged unless the patient gives permission. If he does give permission, it should be obtained in writing and, if a legal authority requires information against the wishes of the patient, such a request should be made formally through a magistrate or other court. If there is any doubt in the doctor's mind, he should consult his medical defence organization first.

When a court report or other formal submission is required for legal purposes, it is essential for the doctor to have a clear idea of its purpose and of his contribution to it. Such a report should always have a clear, factual basis and any opinion or recommendation expressed should follow from the facts recorded.

Criminal Responsibility

Arguments about criminal responsibility have become very much less valid since the abolition of the death penalty for murder and the passing of the Homicide Act (1967), which provided that a person could be convicted of manslaughter if he had a mental abnormality that substantially impaired his mental responsibility. In such cases, the judge is free to pass sentence or advise treatment based on the medical evidence he has received (Gibbens 1975a).

For some offences there is no question of pleading diminished responsibility; for example, a driver is always responsible for what happens when he is driving. However, in some circumstances, e.g. hypoglycaemic confusional states, the medical evidence may be very important in preventing a person from being successfully prosecuted.

Offences Against Property

Shoplifting

The crime of shoplifting has shown some of the characteristics of an epidemic since the movement towards supermarkets began in the 1960s. Open display and self-service present considerable temptation to many people, and since the purpose of such selling methods is to induce customers to accumulate items passively in their shopping trolleys, it should really be no surprise to us when they fill their pockets and bags as well.

Shoplifters include professionals who take orders for the goods that they steal, teenagers who are conforming to peer group norms, and a significant number of foreign-born women ranging from au pairs to the wives of oil sheikhs. However, the group that has attracted the most interest is that of native-born middle-aged women who have been found to have a significant amount of physical and mental ill-health. In one series of 500 women appearing before the courts, about one-third had a history of major physical or mental disability and, at 10-year follow-up as a group, their hospital admission rate was about three times the national admission rate for women of the same age (Gibbens 1975b). Sometimes the offence is a prodromal symptom of a depressive illness or possibly precipitates it, but in other cases it is a manifestation of neurotic disturbance which may be of a particularly difficult kind to help. These women, often the wives of successful men, have reached the end of their time in the maternal role and are facing a major readjustment problem. Psychotherapy is indicated in such situations and they may need considerable support in coping with the stigma which they have incurred in their community.

Arson

Arson is a very serious offence. It may endanger lives, and once a person has embarked on a path of arson there is a strong likelihood that he will repeat the offence. Not infrequently, arsonists are of subnormal or marginal intelligence, but to neurotic cripples with poor self-esteem the act of arson may represent the only outlet for any capacity to feel power over their environment. These are very dangerous people who are particularly likely to respond to stressful situations by a repetition of their offence.

Subnormal patients are usually already under the general supervision of a specialist in subnormality, but if arson is suspected, an urgent psychiatric assessment is indicated.

Offences Against The Person

Domestic Violence

Violence occurring within the context of the home or of a close relationship is probably the commonest kind; certainly murderers are usually known to their victims. It is likely that the potential for violence is within us all and the suppression of that potential is one aspect of child-rearing by which we place great store.

The capacity of young humans to produce major violence is a theme which occurs in literature, such as Golding's horrific tale *Lord of the Flies*, and in real life, e.g. the case of Mary Bell. It seems to occur pathologically when there has been a breakdown in the normal 'civilizing' influences, both within and outside the home. However, a considerable amount of overt physical aggression is not unusual in adolescent males and is institutionalized in rugby and football as well as university 'rag days'. The extent to which females are exempt from this trait is unclear, and the issue takes us straight into the nature/nurture argument to which there is no clear answer. It is suggested that the breakdown of traditional male/female stereotypes is leading to girls being involved to a much greater extent in male pattern violent delinquency.

'Inheritance' of Violence

The capacity to show patience and affection seems to depend to a large extent on modelling on one's own parents and other important adults. It is common to find that child- and wife-beaters are themselves repeating a pattern of behaviour from their own early experience. Sexual violence is usually related to a similar failure to develop tender physical communication with the opposite sex and is likely to be a manifestation of severely disturbed intrafamily relationships. The extent to which violence within a relationship is collusive is debatable and, certainly in my experience, the woman's returning to her husband has more to do with having no other means of support or place to go than with a wish to be beaten up.

The 'inheritance' of violent modes of expression is a major social problem which has no respect for class. To what extent the increasing concern for battered children and wives is due to a real increase in the amount of battering or to a reduced tolerance by society in general and by women in particular is unclear. It is clear that alcohol plays a central role and that the extent of alcoholism is increasing.

The Role of Primary Care

Everyday primary care is concerned with general support, particularly through the social worker and health worker. Primary prevention is a long-term strategy based on continuing social work, support, building up relationships which can be used during times of stress, effective family planning and abortion facilities and better housing and job opportunities.

The general practitioner's involvement from the legal point of view is likely to arise over issues of child care, divorce or marital assault, and as he is likely to have the whole family on his list this can be a difficult situation. Children should have absolute priority, and any suspicion of their abuse should lead to the involvement of the paediatrician and social worker department if it cannot be handled at a primary care level.

One condition that is particularly difficult to deal with is that of morbid jealousy (the Othello syndrome) which may result in murder. Complete separation of the couple may be the only way to prevent this outcome.

In cases of violence occurring outside a marital relationship, formal psychiatric reports are usually sought.

Suicide

Suicide may be at once an act of self-directed violence, destroying the individual, and simultaneously an act of aggression against others. There are probably few of us who have not pondered it on occasions and in the community at large there are many who have made attempts.

Successful Suicide

Successful consummated suicide is 'positively correlated with male sex, increasing age, widowhood, single and divorced state, childlessness, high density of population, residence in large towns, a high standard of living, economic crisis, alcohol consumption, history of a broken home in childhood, mental disorder and physical illness' (Stengel 1964).

The earliest work on the epidemiology of suicide was the remarkably sophisticated study by the French sociologist Durkheim (1975), which led him to the belief that suicide could only be understood in the context of the society in which the individual was living. Durkheim felt that suicide was inevitable in any society, but that it would be more likely to occur when the social structure was faulty and particularly when the decline of religious and social codes led to a failure of a group to control the individual through supporting him—the so-called anomic suicide. Durkheim also described egotistical suicide as being that which occurred when the individual had no concern for the group, and altruistic suicide, such as that of Captain Oates, when it is a sacrifice to maintain the continuity of the group.

From the clinical point of view, most deviant personalities of all types are more likely to commit suicide and, in particular, depressives and schizophrenics are high risk groups. Patients in profound states of depression may feel overwhelming guilt which drives them to self-destruction whilst schizophrenics may, on occasion, carry out their action in response to their voices. A high proportion of depressive suicides have seen their doctor a week or two before killing themselves.

Organized religion has regarded suicide as a crime since the Middle Ages, and this view was absorbed into English law which made suicidal attempts into criminal offences. However, this was not consistently implemented, and coroners had a tendency to record verdicts of the balance of the mind being disturbed in order to avoid religious sanctions on burial and consequent distress to the family of the deceased. As a result of the Suicide Act of 1961, attempted suicide ceased to be a misdemeanour, although aiding and abetting a suicide remains a criminal offence.

Parasuicide

Whilst the annual numbers of successful suicides in England and Wales have declined from about 8,000 to 5,000 in the past 10 to 15 years, the numbers of attempted suicides or parasuicides have increased dramatically, so that these patients now account for a considerable proportion of all acute admissions to medical units. Whilst undoubtedly many 'overdoses' are cries for help, some are serious attempts that are unsuccessful and, similarly, some successful suicides are cries for help that go wrong. It is a mistake to believe that if a person tells somebody that he is going to kill himself, he will not do it, because such people sometimes do. Only a small proportion of people who kill themselves leave a suicide note.

Whether the decline in the number of successful suicides can be attributed to the change in domestic gas supplies to natural gas or to the efforts of the Samaritans' Counselling Service is unclear, but the commonest method now is an overdose of medicines or tablets. Certainly for many lonely people undergoing a life crisis, the availability of a sympathetic Samaritan who will listen and befriend is an invaluable service. However, for those suffering from clinical depression, effective treatment is urgent, this being one of the few psychiatric emergencies where intervention can have a major impact on mortality.

Delinquency

Sex differences in the behaviour disorders for which children are brought to court are evident from an early age. Among children committed to the care of the local authorities, half the boys but only 13 per cent of the girls under 14 years of age have committed offences (Gibbens 1975b). When girls do commit offences they are likely to be much more disturbed than boys for whom some degree of adolescent delinquency is commonplace.

Most girls taken into care are said to be in need of care and control after running away repeatedly from home or being sexually promiscuous—a category of behaviour which becomes increasingly difficult to define. Gibbens makes the point that, culturally, women are expected to be much more home-based than men, and the absence of alternatives for them leads to rapid social deterioration when they do leave home; thus many drift into prostitution.

Prostitution

Prostitution itself is not an offence, but soliciting is and women may be sent to prison after two warnings. About one third of women in prison are, or have been, prostitutes at some time, and it seems that prostitution in women is to some extent a psychopathological equivalent to crime in men. However, it also represents a way of earning a living when there may be no other, and the women are often under the control of a pimp who is usually a man. There is little doubt that prostitutes are victims of exploitation and of traditional views of sexuality, and it is difficult to see what point there is in incarcerating them.

Preparing Reports for the Court

The essence of a good report is that it should present a chronological historical account of the patient's background, together with a short and precise interpretation of the medical findings, including psychiatric symptoms, and avoiding medical jargon. It should then proceed to make some sense of the present situation in terms of the patient's personal history and medical case

Table 15. Details required in the preparation of reports for the court.

Name

Address

Date of birth

Sex

Single/married

Present offence/problem
   Charge (if applicable)
   Court of appearance

Previous offence(s) (if applicable)

Family history

Personal history
   Including attitude to offences and account of the circumstances of the offences

Examination
   Mental state
   Personality
   Intelligence
   Physical fitness

Diagnosis

Recommendation
   e.g. whether suffering from mental disorder, whether anything can be done to help/placement/responsibility and fitness to plead, etc.

without stepping outside the bounds of reality or entering into the realms of conjecture. Table 15 provides a useful skeleton.

References

Durkheim, E., *Suicide, A Study in Sociology*, Routledge and Kegan Paul, London, 1975.

Gibbens, T. C. N., Medicine and Crime, in *Contemporary Psychiatry: Selected Reviews from the British Journal of Hospital Medicine*, (Trevor Silverstone and Brian Barraclough, Eds), Headley Bros, Ashford, 1975a.

Gibbens, T. C. N., Female offenders, in *Contemporary Psychiatry: Selected Reviews from the British Journal of Hospital Medicine*, (Trevor Silverstone and Brian Barraclough, Eds), Headley Bros, Ashford, 1975b.

Stengel, E., *Suicide and Attempted Suicide*, Pelican, Harmondsworth, 1964.

12. Symptomatic Psychiatry

The complex interaction between physical and mental states is one that has fascinated man throughout the ages. The occurrence of such sayings in everyday usage as 'she gives me a bellyache', 'he's a pain in the arse' or 'she died of a broken heart' bears witness to the strongly held belief that interpersonal interactions can have physical consequences. Research has confirmed both the direct and indirect effect of physical illness on mental state. While some pundits appear to hold the view that all mental disturbances are social in origin and others that they are ultimately cellular or genetic, biological problems to be resolved by more basic research in biochemistry and physiology, we have increasingly come to accept a holistic view that takes account of both the patient and his illness.

Bearing this in mind, it is convenient to categorize symptomatic disorders according to the supposed predominant aetiology, and for this purpose there are five main groups:

1. Psychological reactions to physical illness.

2. Physical illness causing mental disturbance directly (brain disease).

3. Physical illness causing mental disturbance indirectly (other somatic disease).

4. Iatrogenic syndromes.

5. Psychological disturbances causing physical symptoms (psychosomatic disorders).

Reactions to Physical Illness

Any illness which impairs the capacity to enjoy everyday life is a potential source of mental disorder. The response of a patient to his illness is dependent upon the severity of the illness in terms of disability and disruption of normal life and the patient's personality, character and social milieu. This seems a fairly obvious statement, but the difficulty arises in understanding the significance of an illness to an individual patient. It has been suggested that disabling disease poses more of a threat to men and disfiguring disease to women, although this simplistic view of sexual difference must surely be particularly unsound during the current revolution in sex role expectation.

The speed of onset of a condition and its management by medical and nursing advisors and those around the patient can be very important in determining whether he adapts successfully to it or succumbs to fear and emotional decompensation. Perhaps it is in this area that we have most to do in becoming sensitized to detecting patients' fears, both directly and non-verbally, and in dealing with them adequately, rather than avoiding them. Social and cultural values affect the impact of an illness, both in terms of thresholds of pain and complaint and also of the support systems of a community or subculture that are enlisted when a member is sick. The lack of such support feeds back upon the patient's threshold of fear and adaptation.

Adaptation

All major illness poses a threat to a person's sense of self, awaking realistic fears about the continuation of life itself, and anxiety is a normal response. Depression may occur when the impairment is felt as a loss, and this is especially likely following amputation of a breast or limb. Healthy adaptation involves many of the psychological tasks of a bereavement and if a person is unable to face the pain of adaptation, he will make use of one or more of his customary defence mechanisms. Denial is perhaps most commonly met and it is not uncommon for a patient to blame his doctor for failing to treat him successfully.

It is sometimes difficult to know how to respond to maladaptive coping and to decide whether or not a patient should be disabused of his unrealistic appraisal of the situation. However, defences are there for a purpose and, whilst it is inappropriate to foster them deliberately, it may be only realistic to accept them when a patient spontaneously begins to use them. Unfortunately, it is common for doctors to deny patients the option of healthy adaptation. By talking through their fears and the implications of their illness with them, many patients come to terms with their illness in a way which enables them to see through any unfinished emotional business with the world before they die. This can be a time of personal growth and reappraisal, rather than an unsatisfactory exit from the world with an emotional handicap accompanying the physical handicap in the final days.

Maladaptation

Maladaptation can take the form of paranoid reactions in those susceptible to misinterpretation (or accurate interpretation when a patient is surrounded by a conspiracy to deny a fatal illness which is obvious to him), preoccupation with the illness which is likely to lose the sympathy of relatives and friends, or the development of elaborate sick role behaviour.

Doctors as purveyors of treatments are often uncomfortable when faced with failure or therapeutic impotence. Most of us have memories of avoiding

the personal pain of maintaining an open relationship with one of our patients
who is not going to get better. There is a need for physicians to heal themselves
and come to terms with their own mortality so that they can help their patients
to deal with theirs. At the moment this is a deficit of medical education, but
hopefully the influence of applied behavioural science is now beginning to have
some effect.

Physical Illness Causing Mental Disturbance Directly

The effects of actual damage to brain tissue by infection, trauma or neoplastic
invasion depend on the part of the brain affected. Although our knowledge of
the anatomical specialization within the brain is fairly good, the functional
aspects are less clear since so many are interdependent. From the psychiatric
point of view, the midbrain and its connections, particularly the limbic system,
are thought to be of great importance in the mediation of emotion, and the temporal lobes in the integration of reality and concepts of self, including body
image.

The concept of a continuum of reproductive casualty, extending from slight
cerebral anoxia to stillbirth, has been proposed to account for minimal brain
damage syndromes which might include autism and specific learning defects. It
has been suggested that some psychopaths are to be accounted for in these
terms and the development of obsessionality as a marked character trait has, in
some instances, been attributed to brain damage when it can provide a means
of obtaining some control over erratic mental processes.

Frontal lobe syndromes with deterioration in personal habits and social
graces are said to follow direct damage to the frontal lobes, as well as the
protracted effects of alcohol poisoning.

Schizophrenia-like Psychoses

The incidence of schizophrenia-like psychoses in brain-injured populations
significantly exceeds chance expectation. This assumes an important
theoretical significance, since it might provide clues to the nature of cerebral
dysfunction which underlies schizophrenia proper. The early development of
psychosis is related to severe closed head injury with diffuse cerebral damage,
particularly where the midbrain is involved. Other symptoms which can occur
after head injury include paranoid delusions, sudden moods of depression or
disinhibition and a variety of irritable moods.

Compensation and litigation can have a major influence on the prognosis
and, unless such issues are dealt with promptly, the development of post-
traumatic neurosis with headache, forgetfulness and irritability may become
firmly established. There is a conflict between the need for early settlement and
that of not making a final neurological assessment until at least one year after
the injury.

Affective Psychoses

Affective psychoses after head injury are much commoner than schizophrenia, and may be seen in all degrees of severity in both the presence and absence of objective signs of brain injury. Marked examples may be seen after minimal trauma, and there is little to suggest an additional organic aetiology over and above the precipitation in predisposed people. Head injury often leads to an impaired tolerance of alcohol.

Epilepsy

Epilepsy seems to play an important mediating role in the development of post-head injury psychoses and, whatever its aetiology, it seems to be implicated in the development of some psychoses. A considerable amount of other psychological morbidity may also arise in association.

Epilepsy can be defined as a symptom of disturbed neuronal function which involves recurrent episodes of disturbance of movement, sensation, behaviour or consciousness. In the past epilepsy was considered to be a major psychosis, along with schizophrenia and manic depressive illness, and the sufferers, whilst sometimes being regarded as in some way sacred, have generally been stigmatized.

The mental disorders associated with epilepsy can be divided into: the peri-ictal, including the phenomena of an impending attack; the ictal, including the bizarre mental content of some attacks; and the interictal, being the effects on personality and emotional development (Table 16).

Table 16. The mental disorders of epilepsy.

Peri-ictal	Premonitory sensations, aura etc., abnormal mood and behaviour before and after attack
Ictal	Aggressive behaviour, disorders of perception including unreality feelings, deja vu, occasional automatism, confusion, focal symptoms including paraesthesiae of the limbs
Interictal	Aggressiveness, slowness in thinking, perseveration, circumstantiality, servility, religiosity, explosiveness, irritability, hypochondriasis.

The mechanism of aura production is not well understood and its extent varies from patient to patient. In some patients convulsions are heralded by a deterioration in behaviour and resulting interpersonal crises at home or at work.

Modern therapeutics have gone a long way in minimizing the impact of epilepsy in strictly functional terms, but major problems of adjustment remain. Society is very intolerant of epileptics and they have difficulty in finding work. It is understandable that over the years they may become bitter. Matters are not helped by the interference with learning that occurs in children with epilepsy as a result of poor concentration caused by the condition, the sedative effect of their medication and frequent absences from school. Epileptics are over-represented in the prison population and amongst suicides.

The significance of temporal lobe malfunction in epileptic syndromes has been the subject of much debate. It is generally believed that if there is temporal lobe involvement, there is an increased risk of personality disorder. Patients with longstanding temporal lobe epilepsy may develop psychotic states resembling schizophrenia with paranoid ideas of a religious nature, ideas of influence, auditory hallucinations and often frank thought disorder.

Physical Illness Causing Mental Disturbance Indirectly

A number of conditions which are not primarily disturbances of brain function can have a profound effect on the mental state. These are usually of an endocrine or metabolic nature but also include connective tissue disorders.

Adrenal Syndromes

Excessive glucocorticoids not infrequently cause mental disturbance, and this can be equally true for the administration of natural or synthetic substances. The symptoms that usually occur are those of depression and irritability, but occasionally there may be a full blown psychosis with hallucinations and paranoid delusions, euphoria or frank mania. When symptoms are caused by hyperadrenalism, hospital admission and endocrine work-up is indicated. When they are the result of therapy, they usually subside within a week or two of withdrawal of the preparation.

Thyroid Disorder

Hyperthyroidism is not uncommonly accompanied by symptoms which can be difficult to distinguish from an anxiety state—anxiety itself, irritability and emotional lability. However, the symptoms which are most likely to indicate hyperthyroidism are:

1. A preference for cold weather.
2. Increased appetite.
3. Weight loss.
4. Excessive sweating.

If all of these are absent, hyperthyroidism is unlikely.

Acute thyrotoxicosis is characterized by the sudden development of symptoms of hyperthyroidism, which may include diarrhoea, confusion, marked tremor, severe restlessness, cardiac arrhythmias and psychosis. This condition requires prompt hospital management.

Hypothyroidism can produce a picture of organic stupor with confusion and paranoid delusions. However, this is an end point and before this is reached the condition can have been developing for a year or two with increasing symptoms of loss of energy and libido, nervousness and irritability, hoarseness of voice and intolerance of cold. These patients are not uncommonly regarded as 'neurotic' until a fairly late stage is reached. Treatment consists of hormone replacement which should be introduced cautiously under supervision, particularly in older patients in whom heart failure may be precipitated.

Vitamin Deficiency

Vitamin B deficiencies are especially likely to cause psychiatric syndromes in which confusion and impaired intellectual functioning are prominent. Malnutrition arising from self-neglect, alcoholism, underlying malignancy or a malabsorption syndrome are the usual causes. Management consists of replacement therapy and attention to the underlying cause.

Systemic Lupus Erythematosus

Systemic lupus erythematosus is a connective tissue disorder in which lesions may occur in any part of the body, including the brain. Psychiatric disturbance is not uncommon and may include confusion, disturbed memory, disorientation, auditory hallucinations, paranoid delusions and depression. It can be difficult to decide whether the symptoms are caused by the disorder or by its treatment which may include steroids. The occurrence of psychiatric symptoms indicates the need for reassessment.

Iatrogenic Syndromes

Illich has claimed that medical treatment is now a major cause of ill health (Illich 1975). Certainly many of the commonly used drugs in medicine can have undesirable psychiatric effects. These drugs are considered now, with the exception of psychiatric treatments themselves which are discussed in Chapter 15.

Antihypertensive Drugs

Depression is a common side effect of antihypertensive medications, probably through their effect on neurotransmitters and their stores. Rauwolfia (reserpine), adrenergic blocking agents (guanethidine, bethanidine, and debrisoquine) and methyldopa all have this effect, although the ganglion blockers (e.g. hexamethonium and mecamylamine) do not. However, mecamylamine can cause confusion and hallucinations. The newer antihypertensive drugs, e.g. the β blockers, do not appear to have these effects.

Antituberculosis Drugs

Isoniazid can cause a toxic psychosis characterized by anxiety, confusion, paranoid delusions, auditory and visual hallucinations and memory impairment. It may occasionally induce an encephalopathy or myelopathy.

Cycloserine can cause depression, confusion, epileptic seizures and acute paranoid psychoses with violent or suicidal behaviour.

Anticholinergic Drugs

Anticholinergic drugs, including the antiparkinsonian preparations, can produce symptoms of atropine intoxication including confusion, disorientation, clouding of consciousness, visual and auditory hallucinations and disturbed behaviour. Treatment consists of anticholinesterase drugs, such as physostigmine (1 mg injections).

Psychosomatic Disorders

There are many physical disorders which have at times had psychological aetiologies attributed to them and each system has conditions which fall into this category (Table 17). Many of these disorders are readily understood as

Table 17. Some symptoms which have been ascribed a psychological origin.

Central nervous system	Migraine
Cardiovascular system	Hypertension, stroke, myocardial infarction
Respiratory system	Asthma
Gastrointestinal system	Dysphagia, dyspepsia, vomiting, peptic ulcer, abdominal pain, diarrhoea, constipation, pruritus ani
Dermatological	Rosacea, hyperhidrosis, atopic dermatitis, urticaria
Urogenital	Frequency, premenstrual tension, dysmenorrhoea,
Skeletal	Arthritis, low back pain

somatic manifestations of stress, mediated through the autonomic nervous system, whilst others are probably best thought of as symbolic (non-verbal) representations to the world about how a person is feeling. However, it is likely that a person needs to have a somatic predisposition (genetic or acquired through experience of illness) before a system can become the focus for the development of a syndrome.

Management

A multifactorial approach to management follows such an assumption of somatic predisposition, and the use of simple psychotherapy, listening, tranquillizers and end-organ treatments all have their part to play. However, a blinkered use of treatments without paying attention to underlying social and interpersonal causes is bad medicine and can only lead to trouble in the long run. It is only recently that we have become fully aware of the poor outcome of gastric surgery for patients with unresolved psychological problems and the same is likely to hold true for other psychosomatic conditions.

Reference

Illich, I., *Medical Nemesis—The Expropriation of Health*, Marion Boyars, London, 1975.

13. The Psychiatry of Old Age

The radically changing age distribution of our population is an issue of the most profound importance for the future provision of medical services. We have hardly begun to face up to it and to develop strategies for the effective care of the increasing numbers of the old and very old who require such a disproportionate amount of our health and social services.

The Elderly Population

Between 1901 and 1974 the population aged 65 years and over increased from 4.7 per cent to 13.9 per cent, and that aged 75 years and over from 1.4 per cent to 4.9 per cent. It is this latter group which will show the most marked increase in the next 10 years, during which time its numbers may well double.

Increasingly the postretirement period is one of several years' fairly good health, and some of the main problems are those caused by poverty when a salary is replaced by a pension based on subsistence needs. Contrary to popular belief, the elderly make up the largest group of claimants entitled to supplementary benefit. In addition to poverty, loss of social role can be a great blow to those who have been active.

Ninety-five per cent of the over 65s live in private households but, even so, it has been estimated that if the population forecasts for 1992 are accurate, 73.5 per cent of all beds currently available for men and 93.7 per cent of non-maternity beds currently available for women could be filled by old-age pensioners (Klein and Ashley 1972). Notwithstanding a major shift in the orientation and interests of hospital medicine, it is apparent that the burden of medical care will fall on the general practitioner and the primary health care team.

The Nature of Psychiatric Disorder in the Aged

The last 20 years have seen a revolution in our way of thinking about psychiatric disorder in the old. It used to be assumed that it was normal for the elderly to be odd, cantankerous and forgetful, and there was little effort made to define any categories of disorder. The elderly, as a group, have poor financial control over resources and, in particular, over the purchase of private medical care. It is therefore no coincidence that the major advances in psychogeriatrics have occurred in Britain since the introduction of the NHS provided the opportunity for interested doctors to work and research in this area.

Natural History

In 1955 Roth published an account of the natural history of mental disorder in a group of 464 patients who had been admitted to a psychiatric hospital during the years 1934, 1936, 1948 and 1949 (Roth 1955). He was able to show that the patients could be allocated to six diagnostic categories with different prognoses (Table 18).

Table 18. Diagnostic categories of mental disorder in old age (after Roth 1955).

1. Affective psychosis
2. Senile psychosis
3. Late paraphrenia
4. Arteriosclerotic psychosis
5. Acute confusion
6. Other disorders

The findings suggested that 'affective psychosis, late paraphrenia and acute confusion were distinct from the two main causes of progressive dementia in old age; senile and arteriosclerotic psychosis' and, in addition, provided some support for the clinical distinction between senile and arteriosclerotic psychosis. Roth concluded that prediction of the prognosis in the individual case on the basis of the diagnostic category alone would 'correctly forecast discharge in more than half the cases of acute confusion, inpatient status of more than 7 out of 10 cases of paraphrenia and death of 6 out of 10 cases of senile psychosis six months after admission to hospital'. In cases of affective psychosis discharge would be correctly predicted more than 6 times out of 10, and predictions for two years after admission would be no less correct for affective psychosis and acute confusion, and considerably more so for senile and arteriosclerotic psychosis.

Prevalence of Neuroses

Other workers have extended studies into the community and towards looking at the neuroses. The prevalence rates have ranged from 8.7 per cent to 17.6 per cent, considering the neuroses together with character disorders, and from 3.9 per cent to 8.0 per cent for all psychoses. Bergmann pointed out contradictory findings with regard to changes in the incidence and prevalence of neuroses in old age. Whilst it seemed from hospital admission, discharge figures and health insurance records that both the prevalence and incidence of neuroses tended to fall off with increasing age, studies of patients consulting in general practice showed that there was no fall off in conspicuous morbidity (Bergmann 1971).

Bergmann carried out a special study of neurosis during a survey of a random sample of elderly people living in the community in Newcastle upon Tyne. In all, 300 subjects aged over 65 and less than 80 years who did not show any evidence of an organic brain syndrome or functional psychosis were studied. Of the 300, only 49 per cent could be placed in the normal group; six per cent had personality deviations which made it impossible for them to be regarded as normal; and 18 per cent had neurotic symptoms sufficiently severe to be at least moderately distressing to them. Eight per cent of the men and 37 per cent of the women had a late onset neurosis of moderate severity, compared with three per cent of men and 33 per cent of women who had a chronic neurosis of moderate severity. The late onset neuroses were essentially depression (two thirds) or anxiety states (one third), whilst the chronic neurotics also included insecure, rigid personalities, mostly with obsessional symptoms, and subjects with hysterical personality disorders, some of whom had shown conversion or dissociative symptoms. The chronic neurotics reported childhood neurotic traits and a poor relationship with one or both parents and tended to be later in the birth order. The late onset neurotics tended to report maladjustment in adult life (marital disharmony, psychiatric disorder in their children, late or never married and of lower social class), or stress or maladjustment in old age (cardiac and gastrointestinal symptoms, physical disability, loneliness, hypochondriasis or impaired self-care).

Taking the various studies together it seems that a general practitioner with a fairly typical list of 2,500 to 3,000 patients, can expect to have about 40 patients over 65 years of age with some degree of organic brain syndrome and about 30 patients with a functional disorder which requires treatment.

The Syndromes of Psychiatric Disorder in Old Age

In developmental terms, the onset of senescence is certainly a crisis. A whole series of major life events occur which require readjustment. In particular, there is declining physical health, the loss of social position and economic independence, and a succession of personal losses through bereavement of friends and relatives that reinforce the inevitability of personal mortality. Loss of a spouse brings with it the prospect of increasing social isolation and diminishing incentive to self-care. It is against this background that the psychiatric conditions of old age must be considered, and in this context that holistic medicine achieves a new importance in the subtle interaction of physical, personal and environmental factors. In effect, what is required is an ecological view which considers this person and his story in relation to his health status, present habits and future hopes in the setting of his environment.

Organic Syndromes

Physical Disease and Delirium

The relationship between physical disease and disturbance of mental state is one of considerable complexity. It is necessary to consider not only those aspects of physical disease which have direct effects on neurophysiological functioning and the individual's response to physical disease, but also the somatic accompaniments of disturbed neuropsychiatric function. The latter are covered in Chapter 12.

Delirium is a condition which is usually characterized by the acute onset of clouding of consciousness, which may range from slight loss of contact with reality to profound stupor. It may pursue a fluctuating course, being characteristically worse at night or in ill-lit surroundings, and it is always accompanied by some degree of disorientation for time, place and person. It is sometimes difficult to differentiate a mild delirium when marked psychotic features are present, with hallucinations and delusions, but correct assessment is vital to adequate management, which is, of course, very different for a functional psychosis and an organic psychosis of treatable cause.

Causes. The main causes of delirious states in the elderly are chest infections, cardiac failure, urinary tract infections and electrolyte disturbances, vitamin and nutritional deficiencies and the side-effects of medication. Malignancy should always be considered. It is important to realize that, with the exception of malignancy and cases in which there are multiple factors, correct diagnosis and treatment usually results in a prompt and remarkably good outcome. This underlines the importance of full assessment, including physical examination.

Treatment. During the acute phase of delirium, whilst treatment is being started, it may be necessary to prescribe some sedation. Thioridazine (Melleril) 25 mg t.d.s., seems to be better tolerated by old people than chlorpromazine (Largactil) and is less likely to cause hypotension. If the diagnosis is elusive or the patient fails to respond to treatment, domiciliary consultation with the local psychogeriatrician is the next step.

Arteriosclerotic Dementia

Arteriosclerotic dementia is usually associated with hypertension and symptoms arise after one or more strokes. There is likely to have been some preceding symptomatology including emotional lability, failing memory and wandering at night. Personality change is also not uncommon, with a growing suspiciousness, which in some cases is manifested as pathological jealousy (the Othello syndrome), and the development of what seems to close relatives to be a caricature of the previous personality.

The changes which occur are gradual, with a stepwise course, and the patient may only come to the attention of the doctor if the family's anxieties are especially aroused or he commits a social faux-pas or legal offence, such as sexual interference with a child.

Treatment and management. The patient is likely to experience depression, which may result in a suicide attempt, and a tense restless state is not uncommon. The latter is best treated with a benzodiazepine such as diazepam (Valium). Generalized epileptic convulsions occur in about one fifth of cases and the cause is probably cerebral infarction. There is usually pathological evidence of widespread infarcts and brain softening.

The management of these patients can be difficult and requires co-operation between disciplines and regular reassessment. Some families can cope for a remarkably long time with a patient who is, by any standards, a considerable burden, and the family doctor must be sensitive to the needs of the family as well as those of the patient. Social work involvement and family support by the primary care team are an essential part of comprehensive management.

Arteriosclerotic dementia is one condition which could probably be reduced in frequency by the effective application of current knowledge to the treatment of hypertension in the community.

Senile Dementia

Senile dementia is characterized by a progressive deterioration in all aspects of mental functioning with memory impairment, disturbed affect, and deteriorated intelligence, self-care, drive and behaviour.

There has been considerable debate as to whether this condition represents the extreme of normal ageing or whether it is in fact a separate entity. The neuropathological findings of senile plaque formation and neurofibrillary tangles have been investigated extensively, and it has been suggested that there is an aburpt deterioration in mental function once a certain plaque count is exceeded. The extent of the genetic and environmental contribution to plaque formation has yet to be defined.

Dementia usually begins over the age of 70 years and is commoner in females. Early memory impairment is usually present and accelerates, so that after perhaps two years there is very little memory left, except for some isolated events of great significance in early life; short-term memory is the first to be lost. Depression, irritability and impatience are all common and loss of bowel and bladder control may occur early.

Special schedules to assess mental function have been developed and the key areas can be readily covered in the course of normal general practice:

1. Orientation is tested by asking the day, date, month, year and place and the patient's name.

2. Attention is tested by asking the patient to recite the days of the week and the months of the year forwards and backwards and by serially subtracting 7 from 100.

3. Retention and recall are tested by giving the patient a name and address to remember at the beginning of the consultation and asking him to recall it at the end.

4. Memory can be tested by asking the patient to recount events of significance in the past week, from during the war and from early childhood.

Early liaison with the local specialist is important if the appropriate care is to be available when it is required, as early transfer to part III accommodation or a mental hospital may well be considered necessary.

Functional Syndromes

Affective Disorders

Depression is common in old age and, in view of the wide range of settings in which it may occur, the symptomatology is more mixed than in earlier life. It is best to consider the two broad groupings of psychotic depression, including typical depressions which are likely to respond to treatment with tricyclic antidepressants or ECT, and neurotic depression, where environmental manipulation and basic support are more likely to be indicated. With the endogenous depression syndrome, there is usually some combination of the symptoms of guilty and suicidal ideation, early morning wakening, hypochondriacal ideas and somatic accompaniments. Neurotic depression is similar to normal sadness which can be understood readily in the total context and is not accompanied by these more profound disturbances.

Suicide. In people over 65 years, suicide ranks 23rd as a cause of death and the symptoms of agitation, persistent insomnia, marked feelings of guilt or inadequacy and delusions of disease are commoner among depressives who commit suicide (Barraclough 1971).

Prognosis. The prognosis for depression in the elderly, if it is treated, is good, although it tends to be marked by recurrence. Tricyclic antidepressants should be prescribed with some care in view of their side-effects. It is probably best to commence with amitryptiline 10 mg t.d.s., increasing the dose under supervision. Hypotension, interference with normal bladder function and glaucoma are among the side-effects, but the benefits of treatment usually outweight the risks. In severe or unresponsive depressions ECT is usually very effective.

Mania in old age may be a recurrence of earlier illness but sometimes arises de novo during this period. Hyperactivity and flight of ideas is characteristic, and treatment with major tranquillizers and lithium usually results in a good response. However, hospital care with good nursing and supervision is required for the acute phase and to achieve stabilization.

Paraphrenia

Roth used the term paraphrenia to describe the schizophrenia-like illnesses of old age. He chose to give them a separate description since they are not usually characterized by the deterioration of personality which is so often found in schizophrenia.

Paraphrenia usually implies a delusional illness with a strong paranoid content. Auditory hallucinations are common, and the patient may complain of hearing obscene commentaries or of being sexually interfered with telepathically. Not uncommonly these patients have had an abnormal premorbid personality manifested by social isolation, failure to marry and membership of unusual religious groups. The genetic correlations do not appear to be as strong as those of schizophrenia, although when correlations do occur, they are usually with schizophrenic relatives. A strong association has been demonstrated between deafness and other major sensory disturbances and paranoid breakdown in old age.

Treatment. Paraphrenics usually require treatment for the rest of their lives and trifluoperazine (Stelazine) 4 mg two or three times a day often seems to be sufficient, together with antiparkinsonian medication if necessary.

Neuroses

Bergmann's study of neuroses in the elderly marks the beginning of what is likely to become an important field. As increasing attention is being paid to the quality of life and as the post-welfare state generations make their way towards retirement, we can expect much greater demands to be made for help with neurosis in old age than has been the case until now. The short, supporting interviews and the use of the minor tranquillizers of the benzodiazepine group have their place, as does the regular supervision of the elderly by health assistants. There is little doubt that, for many patients, some occasional interest shown by the doctor or other primary care worker is all that is required to keep them from being subjected to overinvestigation of the many minor physical problems that they usually have.

Conclusion

It is probable that the solutions to many of these problems in the elderly lie in social policy and the cultural and anthropological factors that are unique to our society. It is likely that in the future the needs of the elderly for continuing social and economic roles will result in a more flexible approach to retirement ages and a greater commitment to preparation for retirement and provision for it when it occurs.

References

Barraclough, B. M., in *Recent Advances in Psychogeriatrics*, (D. W. K. Kay and A. Walk, Eds), Royal Medicopsychological Association, Headley Bros, Ashford, 1971.

Bergmann, K., in *Recent Advances in Psychogeriatrics*, (D. W. K. Kay and A. Walk, Eds), Royal Mediocopsychological Association, Headley Bros, Ashford, 1971.

Klein, R. and Ashley, J., *New Society*, 1972, Jan 9, 13.

Roth, M., *J. Med. Sci.*, 1955, **101**, 281.

14. Bereavement

With the death of someone to whom he is emotionally close, the mourner faces a crisis. He has to cope with the experience of loss and to redefine his personal world without the loved one. If the crisis is dealt with in a maladaptive way, the result is the emergence of a less healthy individual. This is also a time when new, more flexible patterns of coping behaviour may be acquired, thereby increasing the emotional resources available for the future. Crises may be of two kinds: developmental or accidental.

Developmental crises are those predictable events with which we are all involved at some stage during our lives, such as birth, death and marriage; starting and leaving school; starting work, retirement; puberty, establishing a sexual identity and the menopause.

Accidental crises are those which are not expected and include events which may be considered developmental crises in other circumstances: the pregnancy of a 15-year-old daughter, the son killed in a motorcycle accident.

In stable societies, developmental crises are dealt with by set rituals which are therapeutic, whereas in situations of family or social disruption, developmental crises are more likely to be dealt with inadequately and to have the quality of accidental crises.

There are potentially four phases to the solution of a crisis.

1. An initial rise in tension prompted by the event. This results in problem-solving behaviour.

2. Failure of the first phase leads to increasing tension, experienced as anxiety.

3. This tension leads to a mobilization of internal and external resources with attempted emergency solutions. Novel solutions may be attempted or the problem redefined. Some goals may be given up as unattainable.

4. Failure of the third phase leads to a major breakdown. Feelings of helplessness and ineffectiveness are characteristic, but the person may present with physical symptoms if he is accustomed to dealing in the language of physical disorder or if he has established somatic reaction patterns (e.g. dyspepsia, headache). In this state, there is an increase in dependency characterized by a regression to an earlier maturity level.

Bereavement as a Crisis

The work of grief is centred initially on coping with the intense pain of personal loss and later with the liberation of the emotional energy that has been bound up with the loved one for investment in other relationships. The whole process is made easier where the death has the characteristics of a developmental crisis, for example, an elderly grandmother, who has been on good terms with her family, dies after a period of deterioration. Her death is ritualized in a church service and burial, with the relatives coming together to mourn her passing.

It can be altogether rather different if the person who dies is young, the death is sudden, the relationships are marked by conflict and ambivalence, or there has been cause for recrimination in the circumstances of the death.

Phases of Bereavement

In the uncomplicated bereavement there are four distinct phases which co-incide with phases 1 to 3 of a crisis (Brough 1975): shock, idealization, reality and disengagement.

Shock is characterized by numbness, disbelief and great pain and sadness. Reality is so awful that the survivor wishes to believe that it is not true, that it is an error, a bad joke or a dream.

Idealization. The first stage of acute pain and shock lasts only a few days. In these few days that it takes to make the funeral arrangements the worst of these feelings are overcome. The re-telling of the death and the congregation of relatives and friends confirms that it has actually happened; the personal loss becomes a shared experience and support is given. The funeral service itself in its stark reality brings home the truth and with it the second stage of idealization.

In normal mourning no bad people ever die; everyone becomes transformed and idealized. This helps to reduce the pain of the first stage and it persists for weeks or months, reinforced by friends offering their tributes. Normal activities are avoided and the time is spent cherishing memories.

Reality. Slowly the need to look only at the good memories wanes, and it is possible to consider the less satisfactory characteristics of the deceased. The shortcomings, failures and inadequacies can be recognized, and eventually it is possible to arrive at a fair representation of what he or she was really like.

Disengagement. This last phase of bereavement now follows and with it the ability to emerge again into society, initiating new friendships and mobilizing the emotional energy which has been invested in the deceased.

Symptoms of Bereavement

During a normal bereavement reaction, a variety of symptoms is commonplace. There is likely to be a consuming preoccupation with memories of the deceased, and a proportion of bereaved persons have unusual sensory experiences, such as a visual hallucination or the feeling of the presence of the dead person in the house.

The intensity of disturbances varies. It depends on the closeness of the relationship and the age of the survivor. The most distressing and long-lasting grief is that of a parent for a full-grown child. Reactions to the death of infants or young children are usually much less severe. The loss of a spouse is usually more painful than the death of a sib or a parent.

There is an increase in mortality risk, partly because of an increased incidence of suicide (Lettington et al. 1976), but also as a result of heart disease.

Grief generally lasts less than six months and is not so severe as to cause much work loss, attempts at suicide or total social withdrawal. Occasionally there are more profound disturbances and with these there is usually difficulty in accepting the loss together with feelings of guilt. There is also an increase in suicidal thoughts and actual attempted suicide.

Depression is common with associated insomnia, apathy, loss of appetite, guilt feelings and suicidal ideas. The consultation rate for such symptoms increases threefold in the six months after a bereavement. There is often a variety of physical symptoms, such as tightness in the throat, choking sensations with shortness of breath and sighing. Sometimes mourners complain of symptoms similar to those which the dead person experienced during his illness.

Management

Management of bereavement consists of using a 'here and now' approach; the bereaved person needs to perceive the situation accurately. There is a particular need to identify feelings and to encourage the talking out of anxieties, with a discharge of tension and a consequent increase in the tangibility of the material problems to be tackled.

The primary care helper's role includes:

1. Cushioning the impact, but not too much.
2. Helping the person to cope by clarifying what he himself is saying.
3. Helping the bereaved to face the crisis in a realistic way.

The helper must:

1. Acknowledge the person's abnormal mood and feelings and his irrationality.
2. Show confidence in him.
3. If necessary, take steps to reduce the environmental pressures.

4. Strike a balance against too much reduction of tension (for example with medication) which might prejudice healthy adaptation.

5. Encourage positive resolutions.

6. Be aware of conflicting advice from the person's family and friends.

7. Deal with the situation actively and not by avoidance.

Bereavement is painful to all concerned. Constructive help requires that the helper be aware of his own difficulties in coming to terms with loss and not allow them to divert him into avoiding this task.

In modern society our experience of bereavement is slight. The institutions which have traditionally provided a framework for bringing understanding to what can be the most devastating experience of all, are fading away. In the end we have to fall back on each other for support and members of primary care teams have an obligation to provide this.

Case History 1

An 18-year-old girl's father, who was in his early 50s, was dying of lung cancer. Her mother was in a mental hospital and her step-sibs from her father's first marriage had no interest in his welfare. The girl herself had left home some time before and had very mixed feelings about her father, but now that he was dying, she held him up as a model man. Left on her own to travel some hundreds of miles each weekend to visit her father, she was restless, weepy and full of anguish. Her one wish was to deny that it was all happening. She hated coming to the surgery because the very fact of the consultations was an acknowledgement of their cause.

Management

The girl was seen every week or so for a 20-minute consultation over the weeks surrounding her father's death. The task was to bring out into the open her ambivalence and to support her in coming to terms with it. At times this seemed to be impossible. Her father died, and she coped with the funeral arrangements alone. At this time she became frankly depressed in a more overt way with a lot of weeping and was more able to express her feelings. She left the area but wrote to say that she was returning to normal and thought that without the help she had received she could not have coped satisfactorily with her grief.

Case History 2

A 48-year-old woman whose husband had died some months earlier from lung cancer was depressed and had difficulty in accepting his death. She kept thinking that he was working out in the shed and would come back inside. He had been ill for some time and had had to go into hospital earlier in the year. It was cold there and he disliked it and made his wife promise that she would not let him be sent into hospital again. Towards the end he was receiving a lot of medication and became confused at home. He was sent into hospital where his medication could be reduced and he became orientated again for a few days before his death. However, he was angry at the betrayal and swore at his wife when she visited him. Thereafter, at each visit he cried and entreated her to forgive him. His wife was now denying his death and at the same time was idealizing him. It had undoubtedly been a happy and satisfying marriage, but as the interview progressed and the circumstances of the final illness were described, the woman felt able to respond to an invitation to put his 'ideal' personality into context. 'Yes, we did have arguments sometimes, if we did he would go out into the shed.' This sort of childlike linking of ideas is common. An opportunity to bring them out into the open can be very helpful.

Case History 3

One mother, whose eight-year-old son had been drowned on holiday, often thought he was in his favourite seat watching television. The frequency of this experience decreased over the ensuing months.

References

Brough, W., *Update,* 1975, **11,** 499.

Lettington, W. C., Madden, T. A. and Cross, I. B., *Update*, 1976, **13,** 799.

15. Psychiatric Treatment

The purpose of treatment in medicine is to arrest processes, to restore function and to minimize disability. In this respect psychiatry has only recently acquired potent tools and is still at a stage of experiment and evaluation.

A rational approach to treatment in any specialty requires an understanding of the patient in his ecological setting. This means that attention must be paid to genetic, constitutional and environmental factors as well as to the time dimension, i.e. 'Why has this patient developed this disorder at this time?'. If intervention is confined to symptom relief by chemotherapy, with no attempt to alter potent pathogenic forces, this should be made explicit in order to avoid the development of a protracted patient career of disablement in the sick role.

This does not imply that a symptomatic approach is not justified at times, but that the choice of options must be considered. This choice includes a range of degrees of 'directedness' by the doctor or other worker, varying from non-directive counselling or psychotherapy to quite specific recommendations or advice, especially where this relates to social services, housing and occupational needs. A general practitioner needs to know the skills that are available to him from medical and non-medical members of the primary care team. He must assess realistically his own capabilities so that his patients are managed in the most appropriate way. In particular, he needs to know when to invoke specialist help and how to make use of the procedures for compulsory admission under the 1959 Mental Health Act.

Psychotherapy and Counselling

'If any experience can take effect, psychotherapy has a chance since it itself is an experience'

Kurt Schneider

Psychotherapy has come a long way since Freud first became interested in the subconscious and began to psychoanalyse neurotic patients. A whole range of therapies has blossomed and then disappeared without trace, whilst a hard core of theory based on ideas of development, learning and interpersonal behaviour has clarified many of the processes which Freud and his followers described so clearly.

In general, it is fair to say that insight is an important element in change in people's behaviour, but that insight alone and at an intellectual level, without motivation to change, usually results in a new condition—that of therapy addiction. To have motivation a person usually needs to feel valued and to value himself. Such a person is not usually very disturbed, and this paradox implies that we cannot help those people who most need help.

As occurs so often in medicine, we find that there are three groups of people: those who will get better (recover from a crisis or adapt) whatever happens; those whose lives and the lives of those around them will continue to be a misery whatever is done; and those for whom timely, appropriately pitched help can have a major impact on the future course of their lives. Generally speaking, this last category includes older adolescents who are beginning to mature and people for whom a crisis (marital breakdown, bereavement, career disappointment) has rendered them open to looking at the world with fresh eyes.

The Role of the General Practitioner

The general practitioner, in his role of gatekeeper, has an important part to play in deciding whom to refer for psychotherapy and whom to support himself, which may depend on the patient being either a good or a bad prospect. The usual pattern is that the good prospects get better as expected (unless they are unfortunate enough to have money to spend on open-ended therapy), whilst those for whom a timely referral would be most productive are delayed until they are no longer 'good prospects' and are referred together with those for whom psychiatrists have very little to offer. This may appear to suggest that psychiatrists seem reluctant to have much to do with severely disturbed personalities, but, in reality, such patients can be offered little apart from care outside the community, and that is becoming increasingly scarce. It is probably realistic to expect a variety of professionals to play some supporting part in the care of severe personality disorder, since these people need consistent caring relationships as a basis for developing feelings of self-worth. With such patients, the failure of their experience of being parented has generally played a singificant part in the development of their personality disorders.

A Sympathetic Approach

A general practitioner can help patients with neuroses and life difficulties by stepping outside his normal directive medical role and taking on a much more reflective one. He can deflect the patient's question back to him, listen sympathetically and provide a sounding board. When specific problem-centred counselling is required, referral to marriage guidance or a social worker is the best course of action if the doctor has not developed skills in this area.

Sometimes it is valuable to analyse a patient's interactions with other people in a detached way and to look in turn at the communications between the principal parties. This can suggest options for realistic steps to be taken towards reduction of stressful factors, with concentration on practical matters in the present.

Psychotropic Drugs

Undoubtedly one of the major advances of the postwar period has been the development of potent psychotropic drugs for the treatment of the major psychoses, including depression. The benefits of the minor tranquillizers may be thought by some to be more contentious. One of the major problems with psychotropic drugs is flooding of the market at regular intervals with slightly different preparations. This causes confusion and since, with few exceptions, the new preparations represent little advance on the existing ones, it is best for the doctor to use those he knows and to become accustomed to using them in a wide range of dosage, including high doses when necessary.

The Major Tranquillizers

The most commonly used major tranquillizers are the phenothiazines, but other preparations which are useful from time to time include haloperidol (Serenace) and chlormethiazole (Heminevrin). Some phenothiazines are now produced in depot preparations and are especially useful in the treatment of schizophrenia, where it is particularly important to ensure that the medication is taken regularly. Generally speaking a general practitioner is involved with the prescription of these drugs only to the extent of repeat prescription, but there are occasions, e.g. an acute psychotic episode of schizophrenia, hypomania or extreme anxiety, when he will need to initiate therapy. Here parenteral administration is often the most appropriate (Table 19).

A number of fairly common side-effects occur with this group of drugs and it may be necessary to prescribe an antiparkinsonian preparation to neutralize extrapyramidal symptoms. Orphenadrine hydrochloride (Disipal) 50 mg t.d.s. is a useful example.

Lithium

Lithium carbonate is now commonly prescribed for patients suffering from hypomania or mania. For effective control, it is necessary to obtain blood levels of around 1.2 mEq/l, but toxic symptoms, such as hand tremors and diarrhoea, may appear at doses not much greater than this. It is therefore necessary to keep a fairly regular watch on these patients and to check the serum lithium level every two to four weeks. A normal dose is about 1,200 mg of lithium carbonate daily. Thyroid dysfunction is a contraindication.

Chlormethiazole (Heminevrin)

Chlormethiazole is a useful tranquillizer, especially for the elderly. 500 mg t.d.s. orally is the usual dose, but care must be taken as patients can become habituated.

Table 19. Some major tranquillizers and their uses in psychiatric therapy.

Preparation	Indication	Stat. dose	Contraindications and side affects
Chlorpromazine (Largactil)	Schizophrenia Extreme anxiety Agitation	50–100 mg oral/i.m.	Extrapyramidal symptoms Hypotension Skin rashes Photosensitivity, etc.
Thioridazine (Melleril)	Schizophrenia Anxiety Agitation (especially in elderly)	25–50 mg oral (syrup or tablets)	Extrapyramidal symptoms and rare effects
Trifluoperazine (Stelazine)	Schizophrenia Anxiety	2 mg oral (syrup or tablets)	Extrapyramidal symptoms and rare effects
Pimozide (Orap)	Schizophrenia	2 mg oral	Skin rashes Extrapyramidal symptoms
Flupenthixol decanoate (Depixol) oral or long-acting injection	Schizophrenia	3 mg oral (or 20 mg deep i.m. as test dose)	Extrapyramidal symptoms Possible reactions with MAOI group Possible galactorrhoea Possible depression
Fluphenazine decanoate (Modecate)	Schizophrenia	12.5 mg i.m. as test dose	Extrapyramidal symptoms Hypotension, etc
Haloperidol (Serenace)	Schizophrenia Mania Hypomania	Up to 30 mg i.m.	Extrapyramidal symptoms

The Benzodiazepines

It is extremely difficult to keep up with the regular stream of new benzodiazepines that come onto the market. Drugs of this group are useful but they should be prescribed rationally. Diazepam (Valium), which was one of the first, is probably as good as any and is available in a wide choice of tablet sizes, as well as being useful intravenously on occasion. An oral dose of 2 to 5 mg q.d.s. is normal but some patients require as much as 10 mg q.d.s. or more.

The benzodiazepine group are good hypnotics with the advantage of little danger of serious harm from overdose. Diazepam itself 10 mg nocte or one of its relatives (e.g. nitrazepam 10 mg, Mogadon) is usually adequate.

Antidepressants

There are two major groups of antidepressants: the tricyclics and monoamine oxidase inhibitors. The former are indicated in endogenous type depression and the latter in atypical depression, especially if phobic features are present. It is customary to try a tricyclic antidepressant first. If it is of no use, it is then possible to administer an MAOI, whereas the reverse is not possible because of danger of a reaction occurring between the tricyclic and residual MAOI in the blood.

Claims are made that some tricyclics, e.g. imipramine (Tofranil), are less sedative than others and this can be important in withdrawn patients. A usual starting dose is 25 mg t.d.s, building up to 50 mg t.d.s. after about three days and further to 75 mg t.d.s, if necessary, after two or three weeks.

The disadvantage of patients having to remember their medication several times daily as well as the side-effect of drowsiness is to some extent removed by using a sustained release tricyclic, such as amitryptline hydrochloride (Lentizol) 50 mg nocte. Care must be taken with the tricyclics when prescribing for patients with heart disease.

MAOI must be given with some care in view of the danger of hypertensive reactions with sympathomimetic amines in foodstuffs, and it is of great importance that patients should be given dietary advice. Phenelzine (Nardil) 15 mg t.d.s. is appropriate initially, increasing to 15 mg q.d.s if there has been no response after two weeks.

The role of the newer antidepressant preparations in general practice is yet to be established.

Electroconvulsive Therapy

ECT is the treatment of choice for some resistant depressions, especially in the elderly, for acute mania and for some rare stuporose and catatonic states. It is not uncommon for psychiatric patients to receive ECT on an outpatient basis, and this is an important facility for some people. A course of ECT usually involves about six induced convulsions at intervals of two or three days.

Psychiatric Emergencies

What constitutes an emergency is very much a subjective judgement, and in general practice 'psychiatric' emergencies usually represent crises of interpersonal relations. However, they can take the form of violence, both internalized and externalized, intoxication and a variety of hysterical symptoms.

The few life-threatening crises are usually related to suicidal depression or extreme violence. In the first, prompt hospital admission is required, and in the latter, the aid of the police is indicated. Often, however, the appropriate action with belligerent patients (whether or not intoxicated) is to treat them with respect, whereupon they calm down (the 'hold me back I want to get at him' syndrome). Chlorpromazine 100 mg i.m. is very useful for disturbed patients.

Family Crises

Family crises with which the doctor finds himself involved are best dealt with by listening, refusing to take sides and generally acting as an interpreter and mediator. These events may lead to 'hysterical' symptoms, such as hyperventilation with tetany, in which case the traditional remedy of getting the patient to breathe in and out of a paper bag returns the carbon dioxide level to normal and relieves the clinical signs. Benzodiazepines are often a useful adjunct in such situations.

Delirium

Patients who are suffering from delirium require admission to hospital for investigation, and this applies when alcohol or drug misuse is suspected. Particular difficulties can arise in managing persistent drug abusers who will use the most ingenious ruses to obtain supplies. These should always be resisted, and the patient referred back to his own psychiatrist if the 'playing off' of one doctor against another is to be avoided.

The Mental Health Act

Compulsory Admission Procedures

On occasion it may be felt necessary to admit a patient using one of the compulsory procedures under the 1959 Mental Health Act. Sections 25, 26 and 29 are the relevant procedures for the general practitioner and, of these, Section 29 is the most commonly used. This enables admission for 72 hours if a patient is suffering from a mental disorder warranting detention and observation in the interests of his own health or safety or for the protection of other people. Application for admission is made by a relative or by the duty social worker of the local authority, in addition to one medical recommendation, preferably by a doctor with previous knowledge of the patient. In an emergency, any doctor can make the recommendation.

Section 25 allows for admission for 28 days observation and is sometimes used to extend an admission under Section 29. For this section the recommendation of two doctors is required, one of whom is recognized to have special experience in the diagnosis or treatment of mental disorder.

Section 26 is used for admission for treatment and requires application by a relative and two doctors, one of whom is 'approved'. A patient admitted under section 26 may be detained in hospital no longer than one year or on reaching the age of 25 years, if he has been detained because of subnormality or psychopathy. When there is difficulty in deciding whether or not admission is indicated, the facility of a consultant domiciliary visit can be of great help and avoids unnecessary hospitalization.

Concern has been expressed over the working of the Mental Health Act, and it is currently being reviewed.

Prevention in Psychiatry

It has become increasingly obvious throughout medicine that our emphasis on treatment is probably misguided and there has been a revival of public health approaches, especially as applied to cardiac, respiratory and, increasingly, to gastrointestinal disease. The prevention of disease depends upon an understanding of the limitations of treatment and on the potential for interfering with pathogenic influences.

In psychiatry, with the important exception of mental handicap, there appears to be little scope for genetic intervention. Modern treatments have had an important impact on the course of the psychoses, but the enormous demand for medical involvement with the neuroses is unlikely ever to be satisfied on a one-to-one doctor–patient, or even group therapy, level. It is with this group of disorders that we must seek out the important influences and intervene before the damage is done.

Developmental Approach

A developmental approach to psychiatric disorder provides hints about the areas which we should be exploring, for example the prevention of unwanted pregnancies (contraception and readily available abortion), and consistent parenting and educational opportunity. In the latter the following should be considered:

1. Investment in community development, including good housing, opportunities for creative self-discovery in the arts, preschool nursery education to counteract the narrowness and emotional hothouse of the nuclear family and to reduce the burden of child-care for those who cannot cope with it.

2. The identification of high risk people.

3. The provision of counselling at times of stress, e.g. in adolescence, unwanted pregnancy, relationship problems, bereavement, retirement, etc.

Conclusion

We have hardly begun to explore the possibilities in these areas of prevention. As long as general practitioners have patient list of the present size, there is little prospect of their venturing out into the community to develop the necessary links with schools, factories and the other front-line social institutions which might provide a new role for the general practitioner as a resource person in health education. The opportunity may arise if we resist the current pressure to restrict medical student numbers, and instead seize the opportunity to develop primary medical care as the lynchpin of all medical care.

Index